An Update in ENT for Internists

Editors

JASON A. BRANT
KARTHIK RAJASEKARAN
ERICA THALER

MEDICAL CLINICS
OF NORTH AMERICA

www.medical.theclinics.com

Consulting Editor
JACK ENDE

September 2021 • Volume 105 • Number 5

ELSEVIER

1600 John F. Kennedy Boulevard • Suite 1800 • Philadelphia, Pennsylvania, 19103-2899

http://www.theclinics.com

MEDICAL CLINICS OF NORTH AMERICA Volume 105, Number 5
September 2021 ISSN 0025-7125, ISBN-13: 978-0-323-83520-6

Editor: Katerina Heidhausen
Developmental Editor: Arlene Campos

Medical Clinics of North America (ISSN 0025-7125) is published bimonthly by Elsevier Inc., 360 Park Avenue South, New York, NY 10010-1710. Months of publication are January, March, May, July, September, and November. Business and editorial offices: 1600 John F. Kennedy Boulevard, Suite 1800, Philadelphia, PA 19103-2899. Periodicals postage paid at New York, NY, and additional mailing offices. Subscription prices are USD $304.00 per year (US individuals), $910.00 per year (US institutions), $100.00 per year (US Students), $381.00 per year (Canadian individuals), $965.00 per year (Canadian institutions), $200.00 per year for (foreign students), $100.00 per year for (Canadian students), $422.00 per year (foreign individuals), and $965.00 per year (foreign institutions). To receive student/resident rate, orders must be accompanied by name of affiliated institution, date of term, and the signature of program/residency coordinator on institution letterhead. Orders will be billed at individual rate until proof of status is received. Foreign air speed delivery is included in all Clinics' subscription prices. All prices are subject to change without notice. **POSTMASTER:** Send address changes to *Medical Clinics of North America*, Elsevier Health Sciences Division, Subscription Customer Service, 3251 Riverport Lane, Maryland Heights, MO 63043. **Customer Service: Telephone: 1-800-654-2452** (U.S. and Canada); **1-314-447-8871** (outside U.S. and Canada). **Fax: 314-447-8029. E-mail: journalscustomerserviceusa@ elsevier.com** (for print support); **journalsonlinesupport-usa@elsevier.com** (for online support).

Reprints. For copies of 100 or more of articles in this publication, please contact the Commercial Reprints Department, Elsevier Inc., 360 Park Avenue South, New York, NY 10010-1710. Tel.: 212-633-3874; Fax: 212-633-3820; E-mail: reprints@elsevier.com.

Medical Clinics of North America is also published in Spanish by McGraw-Hill Interamericana Editores S. A., P.O. Box 5-237, 06500 Mexico, D.F., Mexico.

Medical Clinics of North America is covered in *MEDLINE/PubMed (Index Medicus), Current Contents, ASCA, Excerpta Medica, Science Citation Index,* and *ISI/BIOMED.*

PROGRAM OBJECTIVE
The goal of the *Medical Clinics of North America* is to keep practicing physicians up to date with current clinical practice by providing timely articles reviewing the state of the art in patient care.

TARGET AUDIENCE
All practicing physicians and other healthcare professionals.

LEARNING OBJECTIVES
Upon completion of this activity, participants will be able to:
1. Review the pathophysiology and common etiologies of hearing loss, tinnitus, otalgia, adult neck masses and dysphonia.
2. Explain obstructive sleep apnea as it pertains to the adult population.
3. Discuss human papillomavirus manifestations in the head and neck.

ACCREDITATION
The Elsevier Office of Continuing Medical Education (EOCME) is accredited by the Accreditation Council for Continuing Medical Education (ACCME) to provide continuing medical education for physicians.

The EOCME designates this journal-based CME activity for a maximum of 11 *AMA PRA Category 1 Credit*(s)™. Physicians should claim only the credit commensurate with the extent of their participation in the activity.

All other healthcare professionals requesting continuing education credit for this enduring material will be issued a certificate of participation.

DISCLOSURE OF CONFLICTS OF INTEREST
The EOCME assesses conflict of interest with its instructors, faculty, planners, and other individuals who are in a position to control the content of CME activities. All relevant conflicts of interest that are identified are thoroughly vetted by EOCME for fair balance, scientific objectivity, and patient care recommendations. EOCME is committed to providing its learners with CME activities that promote improvements or quality in healthcare and not a specific proprietary business or a commercial interest.

The planning committee, staff, authors, and editors listed below have identified no financial relationships or relationships to products or devices they or their spouse/life partner have with commercial interest related to the content of this CME activity:
Christopher Badger, MD; Benjamin S. Bleier, MD, FACS, FARS; Hayley Born, MD; Jason A. Brant, MD; Kara D. Brodie, MD, Mphil; Tiffany N. Chao, MD; Regina Chavous-Gibson, MSN, RN; Kevin Chorath, MD; Cortney Dable, BS; Kelly E. Daniels, MD; Jack Ende, MD, MACP; Samuel Gnanakumar; Tiffany Peng Hwa, MD; Esther Lee, BS; E. Berryhill McCarty, MA; James Naples, MD; Elizabeth Nicolli, MD; Kimberly Noij, MD, PhD; Merlin Packiam; Marianella Paz-Lansberg, MD; Karthik Rajasekaran, MD; Ravi N. Samy, MD; Barry M. Schaitkin, MD; Scott B. Shapiro, MD; Punam G. Thakkar, MD; Erica R. Thaler, MD, FACS

The planning committee, staff, authors and editors listed below have identified financial relationships or relationships to products or devices they or their spouse/life partner have with commercial interest related to the content of this CME activity:
Andrew N. Goldberg, MD, MSCE, FACS: **Consultant/advisor**: Keyssa, Inc; **Stock ownership**: Keyssa, Inc, Siesta Medical, Inc
Anaïs Rameau, MD, MPhil: **Co-founder**: MyophonX

UNAPPROVED/OFF-LABEL USE DISCLOSURE
The EOCME requires CME faculty to disclose to the participants:
1. When products or procedures being discussed are off-label, unlabelled, experimental, and/or investigational (not US Food and Drug Administration [FDA] approved); and
2. Any limitations on the information presented, such as data that are preliminary or that represent ongoing research, interim analyses, and/or unsupported opinions. Faculty may discuss information about pharmaceutical agents that is outside of FDA-approved labelling. This information is intended solely for CME and is not intended to promote off-label use of these medications. If you have any questions, contact the medical affairs department of the manufacturer for the most recent prescribing information.

TO ENROLL

To enroll in the *Medical Clinics of North America* Continuing Medical Education program, call customer service at 1-800-654-2452 or sign up online at http://www.theclinics.com/home/cme. The CME program is available to subscribers for an additional annual fee of USD 324.00.

METHOD OF PARTICIPATION

In order to claim credit, participants must complete the following;

1. Complete enrolment as indicated above.
2. Read the activity.
3. Complete the CME Test and Evaluation. Participants must achieve a score of 70% on the test. All CME Tests and Evaluations must be completed online.

CME INQUIRIES/SPECIAL NEEDS

For all CME inquiries or special needs, please contact elsevierCME@elsevier.com.

MEDICAL CLINICS OF NORTH AMERICA

SERIES OF RELATED INTEREST

Primary Care: Clinics in Office Practice
Otolaryngologic Clinics

Contributors

CONSULTING EDITOR

JACK ENDE, MD, MACP
The Schaeffer Professor of Medicine, Department of Medicine, Perelman School of Medicine, University of Pennsylvania, Philadelphia, Pennsylvania

EDITORS

JASON A. BRANT, MD
Assistant Professor, Department of Otorhinolaryngology–Head and Neck Surgery, Perelman School of Medicine, University of Pennsylvania, Corporal Michael J. Crescenz VAMC, Philadelphia, Pennsylvania

KARTHIK RAJASEKARAN, MD, FACS
Assistant Professor, Department of Otorhinolaryngology–Head and Neck Surgery, Perelman School of Medicine, Leonard Davis Institute of Health Economics, University of Pennsylvania, Philadelphia, Pennsylvania

ERICA THALER, MD, FACS
Professor and Vice Chair, Department of Otorhinolaryngology–Head and Neck Surgery, Perelman School of Medicine, University of Pennsylvania, Philadelphia, Pennsylvania

AUTHORS

CHRISTOPHER BADGER, MD
Clinical Research Fellow, Division of Otolaryngology–Head and Neck Surgery, George Washington University School of Medicine & Health Sciences, Washington, DC

BENJAMIN S. BLEIER, MD, FACS, FARS
Associate Professor, Claire and John Bertucci Chair in OHNS, Director of Translational Research, Director of Endoscopic Skull Base Surgery, Director (Co) of Center for Orbital Surgery, Department of Otolaryngology–Head and Neck Surgery, Massachusetts Eye and Ear Infirmary, Harvard Medical School, Boston, Massachusetts

HAYLEY BORN, MD
Assistant Attending, Sean Parker Institute for the Voice at Weill Cornell Medicine, Department of Otolaryngology–Head and Neck Surgery, Weill Cornell Medicine, New York, New York

JASON A. BRANT, MD
Assistant Professor, Department of Otorhinolaryngology–Head and Neck Surgery, Perelman School of Medicine, University of Pennsylvania, Hospital of the University of Pennsylvania, Corporal Michael J. Crescenz VAMC, Philadelphia, Pennsylvania

KARA D. BRODIE, MD, MPhil
Resident Physician, Department of Otolaryngology–Head and Neck Surgery, University of California, San Francisco, San Francisco, California

TIFFANY N. CHAO, MD
Department of Otorhinolaryngology–Head and Neck Surgery, University of Pennsylvania, Philadelphia, Pennsylvania

KEVIN CHORATH, MD
Department of Otorhinolaryngology–Head and Neck Surgery, University of Pennsylvania, Philadelphia, Pennsylvania

CORTNEY DABLE, BS
Department of Otolaryngology, University of Miami Miller School of Medicine, Miami, Florida

KELLY E. DANIELS, MD
Otolaryngology–Head and Neck Surgery Resident, University of Pittsburgh Medical Center, Pittsburgh, Pennsylvania

ANDREW N. GOLDBERG, MD, MSCE, FACS
Roger Boles Professor and Vice Chair, Director, Division of Rhinology and Sinus Surgery, Department of Otolaryngology–Head and Neck Surgery, University of California, San Francisco, San Francisco, California

TIFFANY PENG HWA, MD
Adjunct Professor in Neurotology, Department of Otolaryngology–Head and Neck Surgery, University of Pennsylvania, Philadelphia, Pennsylvania

Esther Lee III, BS
Research Fellow, Division of Otolaryngology–Head and Neck Surgery, George Washington University School of Medicine & Health Sciences, Washington, DC; Western University of Health Sciences, Pomona, California

E. BERRYHILL McCARTY, MD
Department of Otolaryngology, University of Pittsburgh, Pittsburgh, Pennsylvania

JAMES G. NAPLES, MD
Assistant Professor, Department of Otolaryngology–Head and Neck Surgery, Beth Israel Deaconess Medical Center, Harvard Medical School, Boston, Massachusetts

ELIZABETH NICOLLI, MD
Department of Otolaryngology, University of Miami Miller School of Medicine, Miami, Florida

KIMBERLEY S. NOIJ, MD, PhD
Departments of Surgery and Otolaryngology–Head and Neck Surgery, Beth Israel Deaconess Medical Center, Harvard Medical School, Boston, Massachusetts

MARIANELLA PAZ-LANSBERG, MD
Clinical Fellow of Rhinology and Skull Base Surgery, Department of Otolaryngology–Head and Neck Surgery, Massachusetts Eye and Ear Infirmary, Harvard Medical School, Boston, Massachusetts

KARTHIK RAJASEKARAN, MD, FACS
Assistant Professor, Department of Otorhinolaryngology–Head and Neck Surgery, Perelman School of Medicine, Leonard Davis Institute of Health Economics, University of Pennsylvania, Philadelphia, Pennsylvania

ANAÏS RAMEAU, MD, MPhil
Assistant Professor, Sean Parker Institute for the Voice at Weill Cornell Medicine, Department of Otolaryngology–Head and Neck Surgery, Weill Cornell Medicine, New York, New York

RAVI N. SAMY, MD
Professor, Department of Otolaryngology–Head and Neck Surgery, University of Cincinnati College of Medicine, Cincinnati, Ohio

BARRY M. SCHAITKIN, MD
Professor of Otolaryngology–Head and Neck Surgery, University of Pittsburgh Medical Center, Pittsburgh, Pennsylvania

SCOTT B. SHAPIRO, MD
Department of Otolaryngology–Head and Neck Surgery, University of Cincinnati College of Medicine, Cincinnati, Ohio

PUNAM G. THAKKAR, MD
Assistant Professor of Surgery, Division of Otolaryngology–Head and Neck Surgery, George Washington University School of Medicine & Health Sciences, Washington, DC

Contents

> A focused history, otoscopic and tuning fork examination and formal hearing testing are the diagnostic pillars for the workup of hearing loss and tinnitus. The causes of hearing loss and tinnitus are varied and range from relatively common age-related hearing loss to rare tumors of the brain and skull base. In this chapter, the authors explain the diagnostic workup of hearing loss and tinnitus, review the pathophysiology of the most common causes, and describe the treatments available.

> Otalgia can be broadly categorized into primary otologic causes and secondary nonotologic causes. Isolated otalgia in the absence of hearing loss, otorrhea, or abnormal otoscopic findings is typically secondary to referred pain from nonotologic causes, as the sensory nerve supply to the ear arises from 4 cranial nerves and the cervical plexus. The most common causes of primary otalgia are acute otitis media and otitis externa, whereas the most common causes of secondary otalgia are temporomandibular joint disorders and dental pathology. Persistent unilateral ear pain and other alarm symptoms warrant further evaluation for possible neoplasm.

> Neck masses are common physical examination findings seen in the outpatient setting but identifying an underlying cause can be challenging. A careful medical history should be obtained, and a thorough physical examination should be performed, which will guide the need for follow-up examination with imaging, biopsies, and specialist referrals. The goal of this article is to provide a working framework to evaluate and manage some of the most common causes of adult neck masses.

Salivary disease may present as pain or swelling in unilateral or bilateral
salivary glands. Symptoms may be periprandial or recurrent and inflammatory. If a patient fails conservative treatment, they should be referred to an
otolaryngologist. If there is no clear cause based on history and physical
examination, sialendoscopy can be performed to directly visualize tissues,
provide a diagnosis, drive treatment plans, and sometimes concurrently
provide therapeutic intervention. Based on the pathology visualized on sialendoscopy, treatment options include endoscopic intervention, Botox,
and gland-preserving surgical techniques, which promote healing of glandular tissue, ultimately preserving function.

Human papillomavirus (HPV)-positive oropharyngeal cancers (OPC) are
increasing due to infection with the virus. Most of the patients diagnosed
with HPV-positive OPC are white men with numerous lifetime sexual partners
who have smoked marijuana excessively. In working up the patient, it is important to obtain an extensive history and physical examination and obtain proper
imaging. Once a full workup is done, it is crucial to engage a multidisciplinary
team in treatment and continue following-up with the patient through post-
treatment surveillance. Administering the HPV vaccine at a young age may
help reduce the increasing rate of HPV-positive OPC in the future.

Based on a review of the most current medical literature, this article outlines
the basic concepts and classifications of rhinosinusitis, and delineates best
practices for clinical diagnoses and the most up-to-date management strategies. Learning to recognize and differentiate these conditions helps facilitate appropriate and timely diagnoses as well as helping practitioners
provide their patients with better counseling and care.

Ear-nose-throat (ENT) manifestations are among the most frequently
observed clinical features of systemic illnesses. The patients often present
with overt findings of head and neck lesions such as salivary gland swelling
or lymphadenopathy. In contrast, patients may present with covert findings of auditory, nasal, and laryngeal symptoms that are less obvious
and are often overlooked. Therefore, clinicians should have a high index
of suspicion to identify the underlying disease. Early recognition and
prompt treatment or referral to specialists may prevent morbidity and mortality. This article discusses various systemic illnesses with ENT manifestations that are commonly encountered.

Obstructive sleep apnea (OSA) is a complex medical disorder with significant impact on mortality, quality of life, and long-term cardiovascular outcomes. The apnea-hypopnea index does not correlate well with either quality-of-life measures or health outcomes, so other outcome measures must be evaluated in treatment of OSA. OSA can be successfully treated through behavioral, nonsurgical, and surgical methods with improvements in quality of life, morbidity, and mortality. Surgical intervention should be considered in patients who are noncompliant with or fail positive airway pressure use. As is true with PAP therapy, surgery for OSA improves mortality and symptoms of OSA even when the polysomnogram does not fully normalize.

 Video content accompanies this article at http://www.medical. theclinics.com.

Vertigo is defined as the illusion of internal or external motion. The evaluation of a patient with vertigo in the primary care setting should not necessarily focus on providing a specific diagnosis. Rather, the physician should aim to localize the lesion. This practice streamlines the workup of patients. This article provides detailed information regarding appropriate organ system–based clinical history and the clinical workup of vertigo. Additional signs and symptoms that can facilitate appropriate referral and treatment are highlighted. Although disorder-specific treatments exist the mainstay of therapy for vertigo-induced pathology is physical therapy.

Hoarseness is a common problem, typically of transient nature. When hoarseness does not resolve, or when it is associated with concerning symptoms, it is important to consider a wide differential and refer to an otolaryngologist. This article discusses the physiology of the voice and possible causes of dysphonia, and explores when it warrants further work-up by ENT. A discussion of diagnostic techniques and the myriad of tools to treat hoarseness follows. Additionally, the role of reflux in dysphonia is examined with a critical eye to aid in accurate assessment of the patient's complaint.

Dysphagia, defined as impairment of the swallowing process, is a common symptom and can be a significant source of morbidity and mortality in the general population. This article summarizes the causes of the condition, its prevalence, and the consequences and costs of untreated dysphagia. The aim of this article is to provide a framework for the general internist in assessing, diagnosing, and managing dysphagia in an adult patient. Basic diagnostic screening procedures and techniques for management are emphasized. A basic treatment pathway based on cause is provided for reference.

Foreword

Learning from Experience

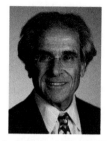

Jack Ende, MD, MACP
Consulting Editor

It is a rare morning or afternoon in my ambulatory practice when I am not confronted by an ear, nose, or throat problem. Typically, I will see 10 to 12 patients in a session. One will be coughing; one will be dizzy, and one, no, maybe two, will report feeling congested. I do not refer these patients. I manage them as an internist should, using my history and examination skills; my knowledge of the disease process and guidelines; and my experience and judgment.

Experience, of course, is essential to effective medical practice. Primary care physicians rely on experience to sharpen their clinical skills. An anecdote is told about the famous hematologist, Richard Vilter. The story goes that one of Vilter's former residents mustered his courage one day and asked Dr Vilter, "You are such a marvelous clinician, to what do you attribute your success?" Vilter replied, "Good judgment." The resident thought for a moment and, not completely satisfied with that response, asked, "But Dr Vilter, to what do you attribute your good judgment?" Vilter replied, "Experience." Still not satisfied, the resident pursued it one step further. "But Dr Vilter, how does one gain experience?" Vilter's response, "Bad judgment."[1]

I am fond of this anecdote and have shared it with my own residents and in my writing as well.[2] But as I look through this excellent issue, "Update in ENT for Internists," presented by our guest editors, Drs Thaler, Brandt, Rajasekaran, and their authors, I am struck by how clinical experience should be measured not only in numbers of cases but also in the range of cases seen. One needs to have cared for patients whose dizziness was due to a significant central nervous system event *and* patients who are presenting with benign paroxysmal positional vertigo and can be managed with repositioning maneuvers. One needs to have cared for patients with vocal cord neoplasms *and* patients with hoarseness that can be managed symptomatically.

That is the major subtext of "Update in ENT for Internists." It is a theme running through all chapters. Common things are common, but sometimes common

Med Clin N Am 105 (2021) xv–xvi
https://doi.org/10.1016/j.mcna.2021.06.002
0025-7125/21/© 2021 Published by Elsevier Inc.

presentations may herald serious and sometimes urgent diagnoses. The guidance presented by the authors will enable primary care physicians to be better equipped to manage the range of ENT problems they will encounter in their office practices.

Jack Ende, MD, MACP
The Schaeffer Professor of Medicine
Department of Medicine
Perelman School of Medicine of the
University of Pennsylvania
Philadelphia, PA 19104, USA

E-mail address:
jack.ende@pennmedicine.upenn.edu

REFERENCES

1. Manning PR, DeBakey L. Medicine: Preserving the Passion. New York: Springer; 1987.
2. Ende J. Theory and practice of medical education. Philadelphia: ACP Press; 2008. p. 151.

Preface

Otolaryngology for Internists

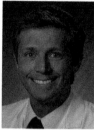 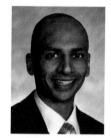 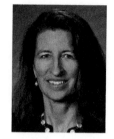

Jason A. Brant, MD	Karthik Rajasekaran, MD, FACS	Erica Thaler, MD, FACS
	Editors	

Ear, nose, and throat complaints remain some of the most common reasons for patients to visit their primary care physicians. The collaboration between internists and otorhinolaryngologists is critical for successful management. As much has evolved in many of these shared disease processes over the past decade or so, not only in epidemiologically but also in diagnosis and management, this update in *Medical Clinics of North America* is timely.

In this issue of *Medical Clinics of North America*, we present the most common ear, nose, and throat complaints that may present to the Internist, with an emphasis on differential diagnosis, acuity, and guidance on when to refer for specialty care. Throughout, the contributing authors discuss standard first-line workup and management. Guidance about timeliness of referrals is emphasized, for example, in the case of sudden sensorineural hearing loss or evaluation of the neck mass. Topics of particular current interest, such as human papilloma virus and its manifestations in the head and neck, are also given focus.

The authors have put together a collection of topics that is helpful as both a review and as a template for best practices in this range of ear, nose, and throat disorders.

Med Clin N Am 105 (2021) xvii–xviii
https://doi.org/10.1016/j.mcna.2021.06.001
0025-7125/21/© 2021 Published by Elsevier Inc.

medical.theclinics.com

Many thanks to Ms Arlene Campos for her excellent work in guiding this project to completion.

Jason A. Brant, MD
Department of Otorhinolaryngology–
Head and Neck Surgery
Perelman School of Medicine
University of Pennsylvania
800 Walnut Street, 18th Floor
Philadelphia, PA 19107, USA

Karthik Rajasekaran, MD, FACS
Department of Otorhinolaryngology–
Head and Neck Surgery
Perelman School of Medicine
University of Pennsylvania
800 Walnut Street, 18th Floor
Philadelphia, PA 19107, USA

Erica Thaler, MD, FACS
Department of Otorhinolaryngology–
Head and Neck Surgery
Perelman School of Medicine
University of Pennsylvania
5 Ravdin, 3400 Spruce Street
Philadelphia, PA 19104, USA

E-mail addresses:
jason.brant@pennmedicine.upenn.edu (J.A. Brant)
karthik.rajasekaran@pennmedicine.upenn.edu (K. Rajasekaran)
erica.thaler@pennmedicine.upenn.edu (E. Thaler)

Hearing Loss and Tinnitus

Scott B. Shapiro, MD[a], Kimberley S. Noij, MD, PhD[b],
James G. Naples, MD[c],*, Ravi N. Samy, MD[a]

KEYWORDS

- Hearing loss • Tinnitus • Hearing aid • Cochlear implant • Sensorineural
- Conductive • Chronic otitis media

KEY POINTS

- Hearing testing and turning fork examinations can categorize hearing loss as sensorineural, where the cause lies in the inner ear and brainstem, or conductive, where it is related to the ear canal, tympanic membrane, and ossicular chain that conduct sound into the inner ear.
- Speech discrimination testing is a useful functional metric of hearing that reflects a patient's ability to understand speech independent of loudness or intensity. It often declines as hearing thresholds worsen.
- Sudden sensorineural hearing loss is an emergency and should prompt urgent otolaryngology referral.
- The pillars of diagnostic evaluation of hearing loss are a focused history, otoscopic and tuning fork examination, and formal audiologic testing.
- Tinnitus, the perception of sound without an apparent external source, often occurs secondary to hearing loss of any cause.

NATURE OF THE PROBLEM

Disabling hearing loss affects approximately 5% of the world's population, with many more suffering from more mild hearing impairment.[1] Hearing loss can have a significant detriment to quality of life, often contributing to isolation, depression, and cognitive decline.[2] The prevalence of hearing loss increases with age, with approximately 1 in 3 adults older than 65 years suffering from disabling hearing loss, occurring slightly more in men than women.[1] Tinnitus, the sensation of sound without an apparent external source, is even more common, occurring in approximately 10% of adults nationally.[3] Tinnitus is often but not always related to hearing loss. It can occur with hearing loss of any type or occur independently.

---

[a] Department of Otolaryngology Head and Neck Surgery, University of Cincinnati College of Medicine; [b] Department of Surgery, Beth Israel Deaconess Medical Center, Boston, MA, USA; [c] Department of Otolaryngology Head and Neck Surgery, Beth Israel Deaconess Medical Center, Harvard Medical School, 85 Binney Street, Boston, MA 02215, USA
* Corresponding author.
E-mail address: jnaples@bidmc.harvard.edu

Med Clin N Am 105 (2021) 799–811
https://doi.org/10.1016/j.mcna.2021.05.003
0025-7125/21/© 2021 Elsevier Inc. All rights reserved.

medical.theclinics.com

CLASSIFICATION OF HEARING LOSS

The causes of hearing loss and tinnitus are varied and range from relatively common age-related hearing loss to rare tumors of the brain and skull base. Hearing loss can broadly be classified as sensorineural, conductive, or mixed (where both sensorineural and conductive components are present). In sensorineural hearing loss, the pathology lies within the inner ear and central hearing mechanisms in the brain and brainstem, whereas in conductive hearing loss there is impairment in the elements that conduct sound into the inner such as the ear canal, tympanic membrane, or ossicular chain.

Hearing loss severity is classified according to an average of loudness thresholds across the frequency spectrum compared with a person of normal hearing. This metric is called a pure-tone average and is a commonly reported measure of hearing severity.

A related but separate component of hearing ability is speech discrimination, which refers to a person's ability to understand speech when it is presented at an intensity level that their pure-tone average predicts a patient should be able to hear—this is a more functional metric that assesses the ability of the auditory system to decode and understand sound (rather than just detect it). Often speech discrimination declines with pure-tone hearing thresholds, although some hearing disorders result in a disproportionate decline in speech discrimination relative to the pure-tone hearing ability. Patients with poor discrimination often complain that they can hear sound but cannot understand the words, which they may describe as "garbled." Hearing severity is often described by reporting a patient's pure-tone average along with speech discrimination scores.

EVALUATION

The 3 pillars of the diagnostic evaluation of hearing loss are

- Focused history
- Otoscopic and tuning fork examination
- Formal audiologic testing

Unlike otolaryngology practices, in most settings patients do not arrive with hearing tests, and testing is not readily available on-site. Fortunately, most of the information to make a tentative diagnosis can be obtained from the history and physical examination, with an audiogram confirmation at a later date. In general, all patients with hearing loss should undergo formal hearing testing by an audiologist. Patients with unilateral symptoms, advanced hearing loss, or suspected to have a pathologic condition affecting the ear or temporal bone should undergo evaluation by an otolaryngologist.

HISTORY

The history should focus on the duration and time course of the hearing loss (sudden, gradual, fluctuating), side (unilateral or bilateral), and presence of associated symptoms such as aural fullness, ear pain, drainage from the ear, dizziness, or tinnitus. The patient should also be asked about any history of recurrent or chronic ear infections or ear surgery. Common ear surgeries performed in patients with chronic ear disease include pressure equalization tubes, ear drum repair (tympanoplasty), or mastoidectomy.

PHYSICAL EXAMINATION

The physical examination should include a focused head, nose, oral cavity, and throat examination with particular attention to otoscopic examination of the ear and tuning fork testing. Obstructing cerumen or debris should be removed whenever possible to facilitate an unimpeded examination of the ear canal, tympanic membrane, and middle ear. Pneumatic otoscopy should be used to confirm proper movement of the tympanic membrane. In cases of conductive hearing loss, there are often signs of chronic ear disease such as middle ear effusion, tympanic membrane perforation, or drainage in the ear canal, whereas sensorineural hearing loss usually produces no visible signs on otoscopic examination.

Tuning Fork Examination

A proper tuning fork examination can often characterize the pattern and side of hearing loss; this is very useful when combined with history and otoscopic examination, often making a formal hearing test more of a confirmatory step or quantifying measure than essential to generate a tentative diagnosis. Tuning fork testing begins with the Weber test (**Fig. 1**). If the tuning fork is heard equally in both ears, the hearing ability is similar in both ears (although there still may exist hearing loss on both sides). If

Weber Test

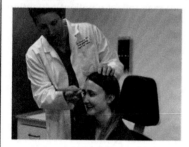

Weber Test Procedure: A 512 Hz tuning fork is gently set vibrating and it is held firmly on the patient's forehead in the midline for a few seconds. The patient is asked if the tone is heard more clearly on one side (lateralization) or if they cannot identify a side which hears the tone better (no lateralization).

Interpretation: If there is no lateralization there is unlikely to be asymmetric hearing loss. If the tone lateralizes to one side, there is an ipsilateral conductive hearing loss or a contralateral sensorineural hearing loss.

Rinne Test

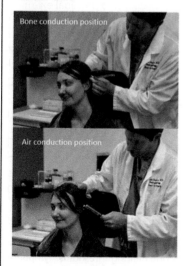

Bone conduction position

Air conduction position

Rinne Test Procedure: A 512 Hz tuning fork is gently set vibrating and it is held firmly on the mastoid just behind and above the external ear for a few seconds (bone conduction position). While the fork is still vibrating (expect the vibration to have diminished somewhat) it is moved off the mastoid and held 1-2 cm from the ear canal with the tines of the fork oriented in line with the ear canal (air conduction position). The patient is asked in which position the tone is heard louder.

Interpretation: An ear with a significant conductive hearing loss hears bone conduction louder than air conduction. An ear that is normal or has sensorineural hearing loss hears air conduction greater than bone conduction.

Fig. 1. Weber and Rinne test procedure and interpretation.

the sound is heard louder on one side, it signifies either an ipsilateral conductive hearing loss or a contralateral sensorineural hearing loss; this is then paired with information gained from the Rinne test to identify the side of the hearing loss and its character (sensorineural or conductive). The Rinne test compares bone conduction with air conduction in each ear individually. In a normal ear, or an ear with sensorineural hearing loss, air conduction should be heard louder than bone conduction. If this is not the case it suggests a conductive hearing loss on that side.[4]

AUDIOMETRY

There are several components to a formal hearing test. All patients with hearing loss should undergo formal hearing testing, which should include audiometry and speech discrimination testing with other testing as needed. Audiometry measures hearing thresholds of pure-tone sounds across frequencies (**Fig. 2**). Speech discrimination measures word understanding when sound is presented at an intensity that is higher than a patient's pure-tone hearing thresholds. Specifically, it removes the volume/intensity component of the hearing and captures a patient's ability to decode and understand speech. It is a very useful metric of hearing that may reflect a patient's functional hearing performance even more so than pure-tone thresholds.

REFERRAL AND IMAGING WORKUP

In general, all patients with hearing loss should be evaluated by an audiologist and otolaryngology specialist at some point. Two specific situations merit special attention:

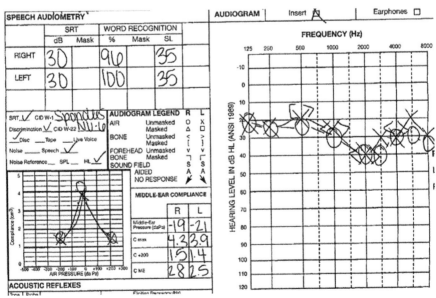

Fig. 2. Excerpt from hearing test showing audiogram, tympanogram, and speech discrimination testing. In this case a mild sensorineural hearing loss is present bilaterally at 2000 Hz. Speech discrimination testing establishes patients' ability to understand speech, and sound is presented at levels higher than their pure-tone hearing thresholds. Tympanometry is also displayed in this test. It measures the tympanic membrane compliance at a range of pressure levels, which can indicate the presence of middle ear pathology.

- A sudden drop in hearing with a normal ear examination raises concern for sudden sensorineural hearing loss. This is an emergency and warrants an urgent referral.
- A unilateral middle ear effusion in adult should be referred for flexible fiberoptic nasopharyngoscopy (often simply referred to as a "scope" examination), as this can be caused by a mass obstructing the eustachian tube.

For patients with conductive hearing loss, computed tomographic (CT) scanning is often used to determine the status of the middle ear and mastoid, as well as rule out or confirm dangerous processes such as cholesteatoma. For sensorineural hearing loss, MRI with contrast may be performed to evaluate the brain and skull base.

CAUSES OF HEARING LOSS

Specific patterns of hearing loss (conductive vs sensorineural, low-frequency vs high-frequency, symmetric vs asymmetric) are associated with different causes of hearing loss. Identifying this based on history, physical examination, and hearing testing is critical to arriving at a diagnosis.

Symmetric Sensorineural Hearing Loss

The most common cause of all hearing loss is presbycusis or age-related hearing loss. It is a bilateral, symmetric, progressive hearing loss that increases with age, typically affecting the high frequencies first. The pathophysiology of presbycusis is a complex combination of genetic and environmental factors that result in loss of the hair cells in the cochlea.[5]

The second most common cause of all hearing loss is noise-induced hearing loss. Chronic loud noise exposure typically affects hearing in the 3 to 6 kHz range, sometimes producing a "notch" in the audiogram, with recovery of higher frequencies. Chronic noise-induced hearing loss should be differentiated from acute acoustic trauma, which can produce temporary or permanent hearing loss from a single intense acoustic stimulus. Chronic noise-induced hearing loss often occurs in combination with (and can be hard to differentiate from) presbycusis. Although when it occurs with presbycusis it will result in hearing loss broadly in the high frequencies. It is usually symmetric but may occur asymmetrically if there is asymmetric exposure to noise (such as firearm use).[6]

A patient with a classic presentation of presbycusis and/or noise-induced hearing loss supported by an audiogram usually does not warrant further workup. Atypical symptoms such as dizziness, headaches, or cranial neuropathies should prompt further workup with an MRI. Rarer causes of symmetric sensorineural hearing loss are ototoxicity (many chemotherapeutics and antibiotics are ototoxic) and autoimmune inner ear disease, where the body's own immune components attack the inner ear (**Table 1**).

Asymmetric Sensorineural Hearing Loss

Asymmetric sensorineural hearing loss is caused by any unilateral insults to the inner ear or brain/brainstem. No definite cause is identified in most cases of asymmetric sensorineural hearing loss, although evidence points to vascular or inflammatory insults to the inner ear in these cases.[7] All asymmetric sensorineural hearing loss should be evaluated with an MRI with contrast, which can reveal structural or signal abnormalities in the inner ear as well as show potentially dangerous tumors of the brainstem that affect the hearing nerve or auditory pathway. Vestibular schwannoma, a benign tumor of the hearing nerve that can grow into the inner ear or brainstem, is overall

Table 1
Causes of symmetric sensorineural hearing loss

Bilateral Symmetric Sensorineural Hearing Loss		
	Pathophysiology	Characteristics
Presbycusis	• Multifactorial, combination of genetic, environmental, and age-related damage to cochlear hair cells	• Begins in high frequencies • Seen in older adults
Chronic noise-induced hearing loss	• Chronic loud noise exposure causes damage to the cochlear hair cells	• Usually bilateral and symmetric but may be unilateral if there is asymmetric exposure • Begins in high frequencies, often a sharp depression in the audiogram around 4000 Hz • Very common in professions where loud machinery is used
Acute acoustic trauma	• Damage to hair cells, cochlear membrane rupture, perilymph and endolymph mixing	• One-time brief exposure to very loud sound • May produce temporary or permanent hearing loss • Depending on cause, may also have mechanical or barometric pressure damage to tympanic membrane, ossicles, or inner ear
Ototoxicity	• Exact mechanism of toxicity depends on toxin • Often occurs through damage to hair cells, stria vascularis (cochlear structure that maintains intracochlear ion potentials), and/or auditory nerve damage	• Often history of administration of chemotherapeutics or antibiotics • Usually high frequencies involved first • Some diuretics also implicated
Autoimmune inner ear disease	• Poorly understood inflammatory condition caused by antibodies and/or immune cells recognizing and damaging the inner ear	• Fluctuating hearing loss in patients with other autoimmune disease • Responds to steroid or other immunosuppressive medications • May have dizziness with hearing fluctuation

rare but is not uncommon in patients with asymmetric sensorineural hearing loss. Asymmetric sensorineural hearing loss with characteristic episodic vertigo symptoms lasting longer than 20 min (though usually several hours) suggests Meniere disease, a disorder of the inner ear fluid compartments (**Table 2**).

Table 2
Causes of asymmetric sensorineural hearing loss

Asymmetric Sensorineural Hearing Loss		
	Pathophysiology	Characteristics
Idiopathic	• Thought to be viral inflammation of the cochlea and/or auditory or interruption of the cochlear blood supply	• May report recent upper respiratory infection • May have dizziness if insult extends to the balance structures of the inner ear (labyrinthitis)
Mass of the internal auditory canal/ cerebellopontine angle	• Tumor at the inner-brainstem interface causes cochlear nerve compression and/or interruption of the cochlear blood supply, most commonly vestibular schwannoma and meningioma	• May have dizziness due to compromise of the vestibular nerve • May have headaches, other cranial nerve dysfunction, or signs of hydrocephalus if very large tumor
Meniere disease	• Exact cause unknown, related to abnormal fluctuations in fluid in the endolymphatic compartment of the inner ear	• Episodes of vertigo lasting 20 min or longer (usually several hours) • Sometimes have fullness or prodrome in the involved ear before or during dizziness episodes • May have "drop attacks," where a patient feels suddenly forced to the ground

Conductive Hearing Loss

Conductive hearing loss is the result of impairment at any point in the sound transduction mechanism of the ear canal, tympanic membrane, ossicular chain, or (rarely) the inner ear itself. Common causes for conductive hearing loss are cerumen impaction, middle ear effusion, tympanic membrane perforation, and ossicular fixation/erosion. These can occur in combination depending on the cause; chronic ear disease often damages all of these structures. History and otoscopic examination can usually identify the cause for a conductive hearing loss, often aided by CT imaging, which provides good resolution of the largely osseous anatomy of the external, middle, and inner ear.

Conductive hearing loss is often the result of chronic otitis media and eustachian tube dysfunction, which may result in recurrent infection and inflammation. The sequelae of this may be ossicular erosion, tympanic membrane perforations, and/or cholesteatoma. Cholesteatoma is an ectopic, erosive focus of keratinized squamous epithelium (skin) in the middle ear space. It can erode into the inner ear, facial nerve, or brain in advanced cases. Chronic or recurrent drainage from the ear should raise suspicion for cholesteatoma. Surgery is usually indicated in case of cholesteatoma to prevent erosion into the inner ear and skull base as well as to stop drainage and improve hearing. Of note, chronic inflammation often also causes sensorineural hearing loss, so that patients with chronic ear disease often present with mixed hearing loss.

Uncomplicated acute otitis media is generally rare in adults, and ear pain is often due to other causes. Middle ear effusion, however, is quite common. A unilateral middle ear effusion in an adult should prompt referral for flexible fiberoptic scope examination of the nasopharynx to rule out an obstructing mass in the eustachian tube.

Conductive hearing loss (or mixed) with a normal ear examinaiton raises concern for ossicular or inner ear abnormalities unrelated to chronic ear disease such as otosclerosis or superior semicircular canal dehiscence. Otosclerosis, which causes osseous changes in the ossicular chain and inner ear, typically causes a unilateral or bilateral low-frequency mixed hearing loss. It is an inherited disorder, and patients often have family members with similar hearing loss or who have had surgery. Superior semicircular canal dehiscence is caused by absent bone over this portion of the inner ear and can lead to dizziness in response to loud sounds as well as conductive hearing loss (**Table 3**).

CONGENITAL/GENETIC HEARING LOSS

Congenital and genetic hearing gloss cannot be easily classified as the other causes of hearing loss due to the varied ways in which they may present. Congenital hearing loss can be due to genetic causes or be acquired in utero. It can produce any pattern of hearing loss—bilateral or unilateral, sensorineural, conductive, or mixed—and can be stable or progressive, depending on the cause. Certain infections such as cytomegalovirus are known to cause congenital hearing loss. Genetic hearing loss may present at birth and thus be congenital or appear later in life. Although likely to be symmetric, it also can be unilateral, and it is similarly variable in that it can be progressive or stable. It may or may not be associated with other deficits if it is part of the syndrome.

APPROACH TO THE TREATMENT OF HEARING LOSS

Treatment of hearing less must take in account the underlying cause, the patient's hearing severity, as well as their social situation. The underlying cause for the hearing loss must be addressed, for which treatment of may take precedent before rehabilitation of hearing is considered, especially if the cause is a dangerous process such as cholesteatoma or vestibular schwannoma. The cause of the hearing loss must also be considered, as it can predict future hearing changes.

Optimizing Communication

Patients with any hearing loss and their families should be counseled to optimize the communication environment by having speakers face them directly and speak in a loud clear voice, as conscious or unconscious lip reading can significantly improve speech understanding. They should also be counseled that they may struggle in situations with significant background noise such as restaurants or in crowds.

Hearing Aids

Patients with more significant hearing loss often benefit from hearing aids. Hearing aids amplify and filter sounds across specific frequencies and are programmed by an audiologist specifically for a patient's hearing abilities. They often can connect wirelessly to phones and other electronic devices. Hearing aids can be beneficial for patients with either sensorineural and/or conductive hearing loss. The best hearing aid candidates have relatively good speech discrimination testing scores. Because the main function of the hearing aid is to amplify sound, patients with poor speech discrimination still report poor speech understanding and have issues with clarity even with strong hearing aids. Patients with chronic ear disease may not be able to tolerate having a device in their ear canal.

Table 3
Causes of symmetric sensorineural hearing loss

Conductive Hearing Loss		
	Pathophysiology	**Characteristics**
Acute otitis media	Suppurative infection of the middle ear caused by viruses or bacteria	• Uncommon in adults • Painful, bulging tympanic membrane with visible pus in the middle ear
Middle ear effusion	Abnormal pressure equalization by the eustachian tube leads to negative pressure and subsequent effusion	• Dull-appearing tympanic membrane with poor movement on pneumatic otoscopy • Often recent upper respiratory infection or recently recovered acute otitis media
Chronic otitis media	Chronic inflammation, infection, and/or cholesteatoma growth lead to destruction of tympanic membrane or ossicular chain	• Recurrent ear drainage • Often have grossly abnormal ear examination; may have tympanic membrane perforation, retraction, and/or granulation tissue • Often long history of eustachian tube dysfunction (multiple pressure equalization tubes, recurrent infections)
Otosclerosis	Bone remodeling process, which involves the inner ear and stapes resulting in fixation of the stapes footplate	• Unilateral or bilateral low-frequency conductive or mixed hearing loss • Usually normal ear examination with no history of chronic otitis media
Superior semicircular canal dehiscence	• Missing bone covering the semicircular canal divers sound around the ossicular chain	• Noise-induced dizziness • Patients may perceive their own voice or body sounds loudly (autophony) • Pulsatile tinnitus • Aural fullness • Supranormal bone conduction thresholds

Less specific amplifying devices also exist for patients who cannot obtain a proper hearing aid. For patients with specific patterns of hearing loss, bone conduction devices may improve function significantly. These devices can direct sound directly into the inner ear and bypass a damaged sound conduction mechanism in the case of conductive hearing loss or route sound into the contralateral inner ear in the case of unilateral deafness.[8]

Options for Rehabilitation of Hearing Loss		
	Mechanism	Indications
Hearing aid	• Amplifies and filters sounds in a frequency-specific manner that is programmed according to a patient's hearing loss • Often able to link to wireless devices such as phones and televisions • Some models have specific tinnitus suppression functions	• Hearing loss of any cause • Good speech discrimination ability • Able to tolerate a device in the ear canal (no active chronic ear disease)
Middle ear surgery	• Restores function of a damage tympanic membrane and ossicular chain with grafting and prosthetic materials	• Conductive hearing loss • Tympanic membrane perforation • Ossicular chain erosion/discontinuity • Cholesteatoma • Otosclerosis
Cochlear implant	• Implanted device that stimulates the auditory nerve electrically • Microphone is worn externally and is linked to a magnet under the skin	• Sensorineural hearing loss • Poor speech discrimination • Poor function with hearing aid
Bone conduction implant	• Vibrates sound directly into the cochlea • Overcomes conductive hearing loss • Reduces head shadow in patients with single-sided deafness • Implanted or wearable versions exist	• Conductive hearing loss (sound sent into ipsilateral ear) • Single-sided deafness (sounded sent to contralateral ear) • May be good for patients who cannot wear a hearing aid due to chronic ear disease

Surgery for Conductive Hearing Loss

For patients with conductive hearing loss, surgery is often considered depending on the cause. Patients typically realize hearing improvement with surgery to evacuate middle effusions, repair tympanic membrane perforations, and restore proper continuity of the ossicular chain (ossiculoplasty). Surgery may improve hearing such that a hearing aid is not necessary or allow for lower amplification settings on hearing aids that are more comfortable. If the conductive hearing loss is due to a chronic middle ear effusion, placing a pressure equalization tube can facilitate evacuation of the fluid, restore an aerated middle ear space, and significantly improve hearing. A pressure equalization tube can be placed while a patient is awake in the office setting. A unilateral middle ear in an adult should make one suspicious for a mass obstructing the eustachian tube and be referred for flexible fiberoptic nasopharyngoscopy.

Repair of the ossicular chain or otosclerosis is performed under local or general anesthesia.

Surgery is often considered for otosclerosis, which causes fixation of the stapes, or other causes of ossicular fixation. In these cases, the main goal is to improve hearing, in contrast from surgery for chronic ear disease where the goal is both resolution of infection, inflammation, and sequelae of chronic ear disease as well as improvement in hearing, which may be a secondary goal. When surgery is performed to treat chronic ear disease, procedures to improve hearing are usually performed in conjunction with those whose primary goal is to address the source of ear disease. For example, a patient may undergo mastoidectomy and removal of cholesteatoma in conjunction with a repair of a perforated tympanic membrane and eroded ossicular chain (both common sequelae of cholesteatoma). In cases of tympanic membrane perforation or ossicular discontinuity where the underlying cause is no longer present, patients may undergo these hearing rehabilitation surgeries as stand-alone procedures.

Cochlear Implant Surgery

For patients with advanced sensorineural hearing loss, hearing aids may not be sufficient. As hearing loss becomes more severe, the ability of the auditory system to decode and process sound degrades, resulting in patients complaining that they can hear sound but perceive it as "garbled" or unclear. This decline is speech discrimination ability cannot be overcome with hearing aids, which only amplify the sound or shift it to a different frequency. When speech discrimination declines significantly, patients may be a candidate for a cochlear implant. A cochlear implant is an implanted device that stimulates the auditory nerve directly through an electrode array placed into the cochlea. This electrode array is linked to a sophisticated microphone and speech processing system worn externally. Although there is a learning period, most patients with advanced sensorineural hearing loss realize significant gains in speech perception and quality of life with a cochlear implant.[8,9] Although there are specific criteria for cochlear implantation, in general, one should consider cochlear implant evaluation when a patient with sensorineural hearing loss is functioning poorly even with properly programmed hearing aids.

Single-Sided Deafness

Patients with one good ear often do not struggle with volume but have trouble localizing sound and listening in noise, due to processing of the central auditory that is only capable with binaural hearing. Patients with single-sided deafness or very asymmetric hearing loss may benefit from any of several of the previously described methods for rehabilitation hearing depending on the situation. If the cochlea and cochlear nerve are intact, they may benefit significantly from a cochlear implant on the deaf side. This restores sound perception to the deaf ear and thus can improve sound localization or listening in noise. If cochlear implantation is not feasible or not desired, they may elect to route sound to the better hearing ear with a bone conduction device or with a specialized hearing aid. Although this does not restore binaural hearing, it does reduce a large head shadow on the deaf side where they previously could not capture sound, and this may prevent patients from having to frequently turn their head to point their better ear toward a speaker.[10]

EVALUATION AND WORKUP OF TINNITUS

Tinnitus is broadly defined as the perception of sound without an apparent external source. It can occur due to various causes, with the leading cause being hearing loss in one or both ears. Tinnitus can be present no matter the cause or severity of the hearing loss. When because of hearing loss, it typically takes the form of a buzzing or ringing sensation. The perceived severity of the tinnitus may not correlate to the degree of hearing loss. It occurs due to poorly understood mechanisms in the brain in response to hearing loss. When the tinnitus has a constant buzzing or ringing character (as opposed to a pulsating or "whooshing" character), occurs in a patient with documented hearing loss in the affected ear, and has an otherwise normal examination with no associated symptoms, it can be attributed to the hearing loss. In this situation, further workup should focus on identifying an underlying cause for the hearing loss.

There are several signs and symptoms associated with tinnitus, which should point to causes other than a central response to hearing loss. Pulsatile tinnitus, which is often described as a "whooshing" or "pounding" sensation, especially when present unilaterally, should raise suspicion for vascular abnormalities. Rarely vascular tumors in the middle ear can be seen otoscopy. Unilateral pulsatile tinnitus should prompt imaging with MRI or CT (with or without venous phase contrast), which may reveal a dehiscent sigmoid sinus or jugular bulb, paraganglioma tumors, or anterior-venous malformations. Patients with dizziness and tinnitus should also raise suspicion for other causes such as Meniere disease or rate inner ear disorders and may warrant imaging and/or vestibular testing. Pulsatile tinnitus may also be due to elevated intracranial pressure, which when occurs without obvious intracranial pathology is termed idiopathic intracranial hypertension (IIH). There is a strong association of IIH with obesity, and obese patients with pulsatile tinnitus, normal hearing, and a normal otoscopic examination should be considering for workup for IIH. This workup may include MRI and lumbar puncture with opening pressure.[11]

Tinnitus may also be described as mechanical or "clicking" and can be physiologic if it occurs due to normal fluctuations in middle ear pressure that occur during swallowing. It can also be due to crepitus of the temporomandibular joint. Rarely, mechanical tinnitus can be due to spasm of the tensor tympani or stapedius muscle in the middle ear cavity.

TREATMENT OF TINNITUS

Patients often notice worse tinnitus when in quiet situations, and white noise– or background noise–producing devices can be helpful in suppressing tinnitus when they fall asleep at night. Any modality that successfully restores or rehabilitates hearing can also suppress or reduce tinnitus. This modality includes hearing aids, any ear surgery that results in hearing improvement, or a cochlear implant. The reduction of tinnitus, which can be quite bothersome to some patients, is often an additional reason for their utilization. The choice of which modality is often dictated by the severity and cause of hearing loss.[12] Other techniques such as biofeedback or tinnitus retraining therapy also show promise as techniques to help patients with disabling tinnitus.[13]

SUMMARY

Hearing loss and tinnitus are caused by a diverse range of pathology, which affects the conductive or sensorineural elements of hearing. A focused history, physical examination, and audiometric testing can usually lead to a diagnosis, aided by imaging in specific situations. Treatment should address the underlying cause for hearing loss that may require surgery. The best choice for hearing rehabilitation depends on the cause of hearing loss, severity, and social situation of the patient. Common forms of hearing rehabilitation are hearing aids, surgery, or cochlear implantation.

CLINICS CARE POINTS

- A focused history, physical examination, and audiometric testing can usually lead to a diagnosis in cases of hearing loss.

- Hearing aids, surgical reconstruction of the tympanic membrane and ossicular chain, and cochlear implants are the most commonly used methods of hearing rehabilitation.
- Tinnitus is usually a central nervous system response to hearing loss, although certain rare conditions produce tinnitus independently.

DISCLOSURE

The authors have nothing to disclose.

REFERENCES

1. WHO estimates on prevalence of hearing loss. World Health Organization; 2018. Available at: https://www.who.int/news-room/fact-sheets/detail/deafness-and-hearing-loss.
2. Lin FR, Yaffe K, Xia J, et al. Hearing Loss and Cognitive Decline in Older Adults. JAMA Intern Med 2013;173(4):293–9. https://doi.org/10.1001/jamainternmed.2013.1868.
3. Bhatt JM, Lin HW, Bhattacharyya N. Prevalence, Severity, Exposures, and Treatment Patterns of Tinnitus in the United States. JAMA Otolaryngol Head Neck Surg 2016;142(10):959–65. https://doi.org/10.1001/jamaoto.2016.1700.
4. Turton L, Batty S. Tuning Fork Testing. Br Soc Audiol 2016;1–11. Available at: https://www.thebsa.org.uk/wp-content/uploads/1987/04/Recommended-Procedure-Tuning-Forks-2016.pdf.
5. Wang J, Presbycusis PJ-L. An Update on Cochlear Mechanisms and Therapies. J Clin Med 2020;9(1):218.
6. Rabinowitz PM. Noise-induced hearing loss. Am Fam Physician 2000;61(9):2749–59.
7. Segal N, Shkolnik M, Kochba A, et al. Asymmetric Hearing Loss in a Random Population of Patients with Mild to Moderate Sensorineural Hearing Loss. Ann Otol Rhinol Laryngol 2007;116(1):7–10.
8. Brodie A, Smith B, Ray J. The impact of rehabilitation on quality of life after hearing loss: a systematic review. Eur Arch Otorhinolaryngol 2018;275:2435–40.
9. Carlson ML. Cochlear implantation in adults. N Engl J Med 2020;382(16):1531–42.
10. Lucas L, Katiri R, Pádraig Thomas Kitterick. The psychological and social consequences of single-sided deafness in adulthood. Int J Audiol 2018;57(1):21–30.
11. Pegge S, Steens S, Kunst H, et al. Pulsatile Tinnitus: Differential Diagnosis and Radiological Work-Up. Curr Radiol Rep 2017;5(1):5.
12. Hoang JK, Loevner LA. Evaluation of Tinnitus and Hearing Loss in the Adult. 2020 Feb 15. In: Hodler J, Kubik-Huch RA, von Schulthess GK, editors. Diseases of the brain, head and Neck, spine 2020–2023: diagnostic imaging [Internet]. Cham (CH): Springer; 2020. Chapter 15. PMID: 32119238.
13. Hoffman HJ, Reed GW. Epidemiology of tinnitus. In: Snow JB Jr, editor. Tinnitus: theory and management. Hamilton (Canada): B.C. Decker; 2004. p. 16–42.

Evaluation and Management of Otalgia

Tiffany Peng Hwa, MD, Jason A. Brant, MD*

KEYWORDS

- Auricle • Cranial nerve • Ear pain • Otalgia

KEY POINTS

- Otalgia can be broadly categorized as primary otalgia (arising from disorders of auricle and ear) and secondary otalgia (also known as nonotologic; arising from disorders other than the ear).
- The ear has a robust nerve supply involving 5 cranial and cervical nerves, which can lead to otalgia in a wide variety of conditions due to referred pain.
- Isolated otalgia without hearing loss, otorrhea, or abnormal otoscopic findings is most commonly referred pain, and the most common cause is the temporomandibular joint disorder.
- Persistent, progressive unilateral otalgia or a unilateral middle ear effusion warrants evaluation for a nasopharyngeal mass with nasal endoscopy and/or further imaging. Similarly, symptoms such as progressive facial palsy, severe pain, or other cranial neuropathy warrants evaluation with further imaging.

INTRODUCTION

Otalgia, or subjective pain localized to the ear, is a common presenting symptom of the head and neck in primary care clinics, otolaryngology clinics, and emergency departments. In a multicenter retrospective analysis of United States national data, unspecified otalgia was among the top 3 diagnoses among patients who presented to the emergency department with otologic complaints.[1] Although some causes of otalgia are familiar, such as acute otitis media (AOM) or acute otitis externa, the anatomy of the ear, its complex sensory innervation, and close proximity to a multitude of structures with potentially causative pathology can complicate evaluation of otalgia in the absence of overt physical findings.

In this article, the authors review the potential otologic and nonotologic causes of otalgia and provide a framework with which to provide safe and effective care to patients presenting with this common and at-times elusive symptom.

Department of Otolaryngology/Head and Neck Surgery, Hospital of the University of Pennsylvania, 3400 Spruce Street, Silverstein 5, Philadelphia, PA 19103, USA
* Corresponding author.
E-mail address: jason.brant@pennmedicine.upenn.edu

Med Clin N Am 105 (2021) 813–826
https://doi.org/10.1016/j.mcna.2021.05.004
0025-7125/21/Published by Elsevier Inc.

DISCUSSION OF POTENTIAL CAUSES

Otalgia can be broadly categorized into primary, or otologic, and secondary, or non-otologic, causes.[2] Although the physiology of otalgia arising from disease manifesting in the ear is self-evident, the evaluation of secondary otalgia relies on the recognition that the sensory nerve supply to the ear arises from 4 cranial nerves (CN) and the cervical plexus (**Table 1**).[3] The source and course of these nerves provide important context during history-taking and physical examination. Thus, a thorough understanding of the anatomy of the ear is critical to adequate assessment of this condition.

In addition to causative anatomic site, the differential diagnosis for otalgia can be organized by etiologic category (**Box 1**). Some entities in this differential would be fairly apparent to the examiner through history and physical examination, such as in the case of significant auricular trauma leading to an auricular hematoma or an ear foreign body. In the following section, the authors review key diagnostic considerations in the evaluation of primary and secondary otalgia.

Primary Otalgia

Primary otalgia can be systematically evaluated according to anatomic site, each of which then informs the relevant differential diagnosis and associated symptomatology. Here the authors review causes of primary otalgia beginning with the external ear and progressing medially toward the skull base.

Table 1 Nerve supply to the ear		
Nerve	**Otologic Sensory Distribution**	**Nonotologic Sensory Distribution**
C2-C3; greater auricular nerve	Cranial and lateral surface of the auricle	Anterior region of the neck, posterior region of the neck
CN V; trigeminal nerve	Superior lateral surface of the auricle and most of the external auditory meatus (auriculotemporal branch)	Face, sinuses, teeth, soft palate
CN VII; facial nerve	Posterior inferior external auditory canal and adjacent tympanic membrane	Anterior 2/3 of tongue
CN IX; glossopharyngeal nerve/Jacobsen nerve	Mucosal surface of tympanic membrane, middle ear	Posterior 1/3 of tongue, tonsils, pharynx
CN X; vagus nerve/Arnold nerve	Small areas of skin on cranial surface of the auricle, posterior wall and floor of the external auditory meatus, adjoining part of the tympanic membrane	Heart, lungs, trachea, bronchi, larynx, pharynx, GI tract

Abbreviation: GI, gastrointestinal.

Box 1
Differential diagnosis of otalgia

Congenital
   Branchial cleft cyst
   Sebaceous cyst
   Epidermoid cyst

Infectious
   Perichondritis
   Cellulitis
   Acute otitis externa
   Herpes zoster oticus
   Malignant otitis externa
   Acute otitis media—complicated or uncomplicated
   Otomastoiditis/petrous apicitis
   Suppurative labyrinthitis

Traumatic
   Auricular trauma/hematoma
   External auditory canal laceration
   Tympanic membrane perforation (blast or puncture)
   Ear foreign body

Autoimmune/Inflammatory
   Relapsing polychondritis
   Granulomatosis with polyangiitis (GPA)
   Sarcoidosis

Neurologic
   Trigeminal neuralgia
   Glossopharyngeal neuralgia
   Vagal neuralgia
   Migraine

Neoplastic
   Cutaneous malignancy
   Nasopharyngeal carcinoma
   Squamous cell carcinoma of the head and neck

Other
   Chondrodermatitis nodularis helicis
   TMJ arthralgia/arthritis
   Dental pathology
   Eagle syndrome

Auricle

Disorders of the auricle are limited to cutaneous pathology and of the underlying carti-lage. In the cause of blunt auricular trauma, such as following an assault or an injury sustained during contact sports without protective headgear, formation of a subper-ichondrial auricular hematoma may cause severe otalgia localized to the auricle.[4] This finding would generally be clinically apparent to the examining provider but none-theless warrants discussion, as prompt recognition and drainage of an auricular he-matoma may prevent irreversible cartilaginous remodeling, resulting in deformation known as "cauliflower ear."[5]

Infectious disorders may also affect the auricle, and clinicians must primarily differ-entiate between perichondritis and cellulitis when an infectious process is suspected.[6] Both conditions involve tender inflammation and erythema of the auricle, which is also typically warm on examination. A history of minor trauma or recent piercing may be elicited. Erythema that spares the lobule (the inferior most cutaneous aspect of the auricle that does not contain cartilage), or lobule-sparing erythema, suggests perichondritis, whereas involvement of the lobule suggests cellulitis. This differentiation will direct management and course of treatment, as perichondritis typically warrants a therapeutic with antipseudomonal activity and good cartilaginous penetration, such as a fluoroquinolone.

Another noteworthy cause of auricular otalgia is chondrodermatitis nodularis helicis, a focal, idiopathic benign skin lesion that is inflammatory in nature.[7] This lesion, classically located on the helix of the auricular cartilage and roughly 3 mm in size, typically affects middle-aged and older men but may affect women. It is exquisitely tender and has the potential to disrupt sleep patterns. Clinicians should not mistake this entity for cutaneous malignancy. Nonetheless, this disease has a propensity to recur, and management of this entity involves a wide breadth of conservative to excisional options.[7]

Additional disorders of the auricle, including cutaneous malignancies and autoimmune disorders, are discussed in a later section of this article.

External auditory canal

Disorders of the external auditory canal (EAC) cause pain through 1 of the 3 CN roots supplying the skin of the canal. Because of the narrow space of this anatomic region of the ear, any condition leading to narrowing of the EAC diameter or even occlusion of the EAC will be associated with hearing loss.

The most common cause of otalgia arising from the EAC is infectious. The clinical presentation of acute otitis externa (AOE) consists of pain and otorrhea, may be bacterial or fungal in origin, and typically follows minor, often inadvertent, trauma to the EAC.[8] Treatment typically consists of ototopical drops and maintenance of a dry ear environment by avoiding water entry to the EAC. However, debridement by an otolaryngologist may be required to clear the infection if sufficient debris is present to limit therapeutic delivery, and multiple debridements may be required early in the disease course for severe infection. On occasion, the EAC is so narrowed from infection that temporary placement of a wick is required to stent the ear canal open and allow delivery of topical medications. Oral antibiotics are generally not indicated in otherwise uncompleted AOE.

Herpes zoster oticus (HZO) is caused by reactivation of a latent Varicella zoster virus infection in the geniculate ganglion and affecting the EAC.[9] It is characterized by an upper respiratory infection followed by severe otalgia and a vesicular eruption principally involving the EAC but may also involve the auricle and tympanic membrane. When associated with an ipsilateral facial palsy, this condition is known as Ramsay-Hunt syndrome. However, HZO may also progress to involve adjacent CNs or additional branches of the facial nerve, causing sensorineural hearing loss, tinnitus, vertigo, taste change, or hyperacusis. Management following prompt recognition typically includes antivirals and corticosteroids, although the efficacy of both have not been assessed with large-scale clinical trials.[10,11] If facial palsy with incomplete eye closure is present, eye care is also advised to avoid exposure keratitis.

Another critically important infectious cause of otalgia in the EAC is malignant otitis externa (MOE),[12] which classically occurs in older patients with a history of diabetes mellitus, although any immunocompromised state confers risk of MOE. A patient with MOE will typically have a more indolent or subacute presentation than AOE, but with similar initial symptoms of otalgia and otorrhea, classically following cerumen removal. On examination, patients will pathognomonically demonstrate granulation tissue at the bony-cartilaginous junction of the EAC. This tissue should be biopsied to rule out malignancy as an alternate cause. Partial or complete facial palsy may be present but is not required. Additional cranial neuropathies may also be present in severe disease tracking along the anterior or lateral skull base. Imaging with computed tomography (CT) of the temporal bone will demonstrate osseous erosion of the temporal bone in the EAC, which in severe cases may be extensive. Treatment is primarily medical and requires long-term systemic antibiotics, often lasting 4 to 6 months. Antibiotic course is culture directed and serial imaging with gallium scan, contrast-enhanced MRI, or PET/CT is used to determine treatment response.[13] The exact role of surgical debridement and hyperbaric oxygen is controversial but may be warranted in failure of medical management or as an adjunctive therapy.

Otalgia of the EAC may be attributable to noninfectious causes, such as ear foreign body. In the older population, it is not uncommon for patients to inadvertently lodge a portion of a hearing aid or ear plug. If unrecognized, this can cause local inflammation and potentially a secondary infection. In children, ear foreign bodies may consist of any material—organic or inorganic—that is small enough to fit in the pediatric EAC.[14] Organic material is particularly prone to secondary infection. Prompt recognition and careful removal of the foreign body is necessary, and ototopical therapy may be advised to treat residual inflammation. On occasion, a small insect is the responsible offender, in which case viscous lidocaine or mineral oil should be used to terminate the insect before removal.

Congenital lesions of the EAC are generally painless.[15] However, they can occasionally cause pain in the setting of secondary infection. In the presence of large size or recurrent infections, clinicians should retain a high level of suspicion for a possible branchial cleft cyst. If a branchial cleft cyst is identified, consultation with an otolaryngologist is recommended for surgical excision.

Lastly, the patient's prior history may yield important diagnostic clues. Patients who are chronically exposed to bisphosphonates or who have undergone radiation of the head and neck are at risk for development of osteoradionecrosis (ORN).[16] Thus, patients who present with otalgia and are found to have exposed bone in the EAC with a history of bisphosphonate use or head and neck radiation may be suffering from chronic ORN. Typically these patients will see a reduction in pain once the active phase of this disease has passed, but referral to otolaryngology is warranted for close monitoring and management of this condition.

Middle ear and mastoid temporal bone

Disorders of the middle ear and mastoid temporal bone have the potential to cause otalgia through both infectious and noninfectious means. Because of the nature of the middle ear as an enclosed space (in the absence of a tympanic membrane perforation) containing the ossicles, pathology of the middle ear will typically be associated with hearing loss. Depending on the exact cause, additional symptomatology may include otorrhea, vertigo, aural fullness, and pressure.

Noninfectious tympanic membrane perforation may be secondary to penetrating trauma, previous otologic procedure, or blast injury.[17] In these circumstances, the acute event leading to perforation is generally known to the patient and will have been associated with significant pain. On otoscopic examination, a tympanic membrane perforation may be visible, with or without associated evidence of recent trauma, such as blood products. The presence of disproportionate hearing loss may suggest ossicular discontinuity. A tuning fork examination can be used to elucidate conductive versus sensorineural hearing loss. In general, no acute intervention is warranted for a conductive hearing loss. However, if there is evidence of, or concern for, substantial new sensorineural hearing loss, or significant vertigo/apparent nystagmus should raise concerns for a possible perilymphatic fistula and need for urgent surgical intervention, particularly in the presence of clear otorrhea on examination with a history of penetrating trauma. Prompt evaluation with audiometry and otolaryngologic consultation is warranted.

With respect to infectious causes, the middle ear may be afflicted with acute and chronic otitis media, both of which have the potential to cause painful symptoms. AOM, most commonly occurring in children, is typically associated with a preceding upper respiratory tract infection.[18,19] On examination, an inflamed and erythematous tympanic membrane is appreciated and in the case of suppurative AOM purulence may be visible through a spontaneously ruptured tympanic membrane. In the case of otherwise uncomplicated AOM, treatment is primarily with oral antibiotics in the presence of an intact tympanic membrane with the addition of ototopical therapy in the presence of a ruptured tympanic membrane. Although treatment is often initially observational in the pediatric population due to the preponderance of viral cause, AOM in an adult is typically bacterial and warrants prompt treatment. Notably, AOM has the potential to be associated with a variety of serious complications, including facial palsy, coalescent mastoiditis, temporal bone subperiosteal abscess, sigmoid sinus thrombosis, meningitis, encephalitis, and brain abscess, among others.[18,19] In such cases, the patient should be evaluated for parenteral antibiotic therapy and possible surgical intervention to decompress the middle and mastoid spaces through either an ear tube, incision and drainage, or mastoidectomy.[17] Clinicians and patients alike should be aware of these potentially serious complications of AOM.

Chronic otitis media (COM) is a broad term encompassing multiple entities that cause long-term otologic symptoms. These entities include, but are not limited to, chronic tympanic membrane perforation, cholesteatoma, and eustachian tube dysfunction. Typically, these entities are not painful in the absence of an acute exacerbation, such as a secondary infection.[20] However, they can be associated with vague painlike symptoms of aural fullness or pressure. Thorough evaluation of a patient with chronic ear disease reporting new pain includes thorough otoscopic examination to evaluate for new infection and potentially imaging studies to assess for disease progression or recurrence in the case of cholesteatoma.

Inner ear and petrous apex of the temporal bone

Disorders of the inner ear—inclusive of the cochlea (the hearing organ) and the labyrinth (the balance organ)—are generally not painful. This generalization includes entities leading to significant functional impairment, such as viral labyrinthitis and sudden sensorineural hearing loss, which can result in permanent vestibular or audiologic dysfunction but are not associated with pain. Well-recognized mass lesions of the lateral skull base, such as vestibular schwannoma and glomus jugulare, are also typically painless entities.

Consistent with the other anatomic sites of the ear, infectious entities affecting the inner ear and medial temporal bone may be associated with pain. One such entity is suppurative labyrinthitis,[21] typically associated with sensorineural hearing loss and significant vertigo, and may be a complication of AOM or a superinfected cholesteatoma. Treatment is with systemic antibiotic therapy and consideration for surgical exploration as warranted. Another entity affecting this region is petrous apicitis, an osteomyelitic infection of the petrous apex (medial aspect) of the temporal bone classically associated with Gradenigo's triad of retroorbital pain, otorrhea, and an abducens palsy.[22] Treatment is generally medical with parenteral antibiotics.

In the absence of infectious cause, new and severe otalgia that is associated with objective findings of inner ear dysfunction (sensorineural hearing loss, vestibular hypofunction) should raise the ominous specter of something atypical, and further imaging should be obtained to evaluate for underlying malignancy.

Secondary Otalgia

It has been said that 50% of ear pain is secondary otalgia, and the other 50% is dental pathology.[23] With the exception of cutaneous auricular disorders, otalgia attributable to primary otologic disease is universally associated with additional otologic symptoms, such as hearing loss, tinnitus, otorrhea, or vertigo. Thus, truly isolated otalgia or otalgia in the absence of other otologic symptoms is highly suspicious for a secondary or referred cause.

Dental pathology and temporomandibular joint disorder

The most common causes of nonotologic ear pain are dental pathology, such as caries or gingivitis, and TMJ disorder, inclusive of arthralgia and frank arthritis.[23,24] Although both entities may be suggested by findings on physical examination, proper management of these conditions involves referral or coordination with dental medicine or oral surgery. In the case of TMJ disorder, some patients with myofascial pain without frank joint dysfunction will benefit from conservative management, which is comprised of warm compresses, intermittent nonsteroidfal anti-inflammatory drug (NSAID) use, and isometric jaw exercises. Some patients may benefit from physical therapy for the TMJ or fitting by their dentist or oral surgeon for a night guard to combat nocturnal bruxism.

Nasopharynx/oropharynx/hypopharynx

Because of the nerve supply of the ear, otalgia may be referred from the nasopharynx (via CN IX and V2), oropharynx (CN IX/X), and hypopharynx (CN X). This pain may be infectious, noninfectious, or neoplastic in cause, and patients who report associated symptoms localized to the pharynx such as progressive vocal dysfunction, respiratory insufficiency/stridor, and progressive odynophagia/dysphagia should be referred for laryngoscopic evaluation.[25] Further, otalgia associated with a neck mass should be considered a malignancy until proved otherwise.

Infectious causes that may cause referred ear pain include nasopharyngitis, tonsillitis, pharyngitis, and supraglottitis. At times, the patient's otalgia is so intense and the feeling subjectively localized to the ear itself that they are hard pressed to be convinced that their infection has an alternative source.[25] Lastly, neoplasms of these respective sites have potential to cause otalgia, through either stretching of the nerves, direct invasion, or mass effect, as in the case of a nasopharyngeal mass blocking the eustachian tube and leading to a unilateral middle ear effusion.[26] Treatment of these conditions is directed to the underlying cause. Although otalgia should resolve with adequate management of the underlying condition in infectious causes and significantly improve with treatment of an underlying malignancy, some patients may experience chronic pain disorder following treatment.

Cervical spine

Cervical spine degenerative disease, consistent of disk changes/herniation, facet disease, and spinal/foraminal stenosis, has been shown to be associated with referred otalgia.[27] CSDD is thought to be resultant of pain fibers in the upper cervical plexus affecting the greater auricular and lesser occipital nerves. A prior history of rheumatologic disease and concomitant or recurrent neck pain are both predictive of positive imaging findings. Patients are generally diagnosed on MRI and have demonstrated improvement in otalgia symptoms with cervical spine physical therapy. Failure of conservative measures warrants referral for evaluation by a spine specialist.

Eagle syndrome

Eagle syndrome is a clinical entity resulting from elongation of the styloid process secondary to calcification of the stylohyoid ligament, often following trauma or tonsillitis. The clinical syndrome associated with Eagle syndrome is variable but includes recurrent throat pain, globus sensation, dysphagia, and referred otalgia.[28] Isolated otalgia is uncommon. Diagnosis can be made with CT demonstrating calcification of the stylohyoid ligament. Treatment is conservative with pain management as needed using NSAIDs, but surgical excision may be warranted in patients with persistent or intolerable symptoms.

Neuropathic pain and migraine

In some patients, otalgia is attributable to a migrainous syndrome in which symptoms are associated with identifiable triggers and with headache or headache syndromes.[29] In such cases, most patients are responsive to antimigraine medications despite reporting isolated otalgia at the time of presentation. On certain occasions, otalgia can be attributable to neuralgia (trigeminal, glossopharyngeal, geniculate, all have been implicated) with or without other more classic symptoms such as hemifacial spasm in trigeminal neuralgia.[30,31] Patients may respond to neuropathic pain management with targeted medications, or in rare circumstances, they may be candidates for microvascular decompression with neurosurgery.[31–33]

Otologic Manifestations of Systemic Disease

Autoimmune and granulomatous disease

Autoimmune conditions have the potential to affect nearly any site in the body, and otologic manifestations of autoimmune disease are numerous. Although hearing loss and vertigo are implicated in a wide variety of autoimmune conditions, otalgia is specific to a relative paucity. Relapsing polychondritis, sarcoidosis of the middle ear, and granulomatosis with polyangiitis (GPA; formerly known as Wegener granulomatosis) may cause otalgia.[34–36] Relapsing polychondritis would generally be clinically apparent, with visible tenderness and inflammation of the auricle that is noninfectious and follows a relapsing-remitting time course. Sarcoidosis may be suspected based on prior history and clinical scenario; serologic studies demonstrating hypercalcemia and elevated ACE levels may be supportive. GPA is similarly a granulomatous disorder and can be associated with significant pain and middle ear effusions due to mucosal involvement of the disease. Serologic studies with elevated c-antineutrophil cytoplasmic antibody is supportive of this diagnosis. However, tissue biopsy from the middle ear or mastoid may be required to definitively confirm the diagnosis in both sarcoidosis and GPA for specific cases.

Malignancy/neoplasm

In rare cases, otalgia is attributable to malignancy affecting the ear and temporal bone, and this may be a clinically apparent cutaneous malignancy in the preauricular soft tissue, postauricular soft tissues, on the auricle itself, or in the ear canal. Treatment of this entity depends on the underlying pathology but may range from wide local excision to extensive surgical resection and reconstruction with postoperative radiation.[37] Chronic otitis externa not responsive to typical treatments should raise concern for malignancy of the external auditory canal, and biopsy should be considered.

Although benign nerve sheath and vascular tumors of the temporal bone are not typically associated with pain, a temporal bone neoplasm with significant otalgia raises concern for metastatic tumor. Previous reports have demonstrated this exact presentation in several malignancies, including adenocarcinoma and breast.[38,39]

CLINICAL EVALUATION OF THE PATIENT WITH OTALGIA

Because of the multitude of potential causes, the authors advise a systematic approach to clinical evaluation of the patient with otalgia. In this section, they review critical elements of the history and physical examination and discuss clinical pearls for diagnostic workup.

History

A thorough history is invaluable in the evaluation of any patient, and otalgia is no exception. Patients should be asked to characterize the "PQRST" of their pain. Position of the pain can yield important insights, as preauricular pain strongly suggests TMJ disorder. Quality may be described as dull, sore, throbbing, or sharp; neuropathic pain is typically sharp and shooting in quality. Radiation to other sites and high severity may increase concern for secondary otalgia. Lastly, time course must fit the proposed cause, and patients should report both timing of onset and overall progression as relapsing/remitting versus constant or crescendo.

Every patient presenting with an ear-related complaint should be asked a complete otologic review of symptoms, inclusive of hearing loss, tinnitus, vertigo/imbalance, otalgia, otorrhea, facial weakness, or twitching (relevant due to the tortuous intratemporal course of the facial nerve). Pertinent positives should be further detailed.

Past medical history should include any history of noise exposure, personal history of radiation to the head and neck, history of head trauma, headache or migraine history, and history of autoimmune disease. All prior otologic history, inclusive of recurrent infections, childhood ear procedures, and any otologic surgery, should be elicited. Pertinent family history includes disorders of hearing and imbalance, as well as history of migraine/headache disorder, pain disorder, malignancies, and autoimmune disorders. Social history inclusive of occupation (to assess for occupational exposures or hazards), toxic exposures, medications, and allergies should be thoroughly reviewed.

Physical Examination

Because of the extensive differential diagnosis at hand, a thorough physical examination is recommended in all patients presenting with otalgia, with particular focus on the most common causes and the most important "can't miss" findings.

A thorough ear examination begins with careful examination of the auricle itself including the anterior and posterior faces, with close attention paid to any discoloration or lesions of the skin, including dermatitis, cellulitic changes, or vesicular eruption. Hair-bearing skin in the postauricular/mastoid region and the region of the postauricular crease should be carefully examined and assessed for tenderness to palpation. Subsequently, a thorough otoscopic examination should be performed with careful sequential systematic evaluation of the external auditory canal, tympanic membrane, and middle ear space. The external auditory canal skin should be evaluated for evidence of dermatitis, ulceration, polypoid degeneration, exposed bone, vesicular eruption, and any other focal lesions. The tympanic membrane should be evaluated for erythema that suggests a current infection, scarring that suggests prior infection, and retraction into the middle ear space, which may suggest chronic ear disease or eustachian tube dysfunction. The middle ear space itself should be assessed, if not otherwise obstructed from view by an opaque tympanic membrane. If a serous effusion is present bilaterally, the patient may benefit from a course of nasal and/or oral corticosteroids. Subsequent follow-up with otolaryngology may be advised for consultation to undergo myringotomy and tube placement. If a unilateral serous effusion is present, referral to otolaryngology for nasal endoscopy and possible further imaging is advised to rule out an obstructive nasopharyngeal mass as the underlying cause.

Next, a comprehensive head and neck examination should be completed. During the intraoral examination, the hard palate and dentition should be carefully examined for signs of dental pathology, including caries, gingivitis, and bruxism. The posterior oropharynx and tonsils should also be carefully examined for any signs of asymmetry. If there are significant risk factors or high suspicion for oropharyngeal malignancy, the provider may consider gentle palpation of the base of tongue with a gloved finger while holding the protruded tongue steady with dry gauze. Lastly, the TMJ should be examined, assessing for subluxation with opening/closing of the jaw, as well as assessing for tenderness to palpation.

The neck should be thoroughly examined for lymphadenopathy and assessment of any focal tenderness. Focal tenderness along the greater cornu of the hyoid, superior and lateral to the laryngeal complex and anterior to the sternocleidomastoid, may suggest Eagle syndrome. In addition, the cervical spine should be gently palpated and assessed for reproducibility of the patient's symptoms with manipulation of the cervical spine.

A thorough CN examination should also be completed. The major divisions of the facial nerve musculature should be examined individually and simultaneous bilateral comparison performed to assess for asymmetry. Gross hearing may be assessed to finger rub if an audiogram has not been performed. If a 512-Hz tuning fork is available, tuning fork examination may be additionally performed.

Critically, if no cause for the patient's otalgia is determined, a nasopharyngolaryngoscopy is necessary to evaluate for neoplasm, as otalgia may herald head and neck malignancy with an otherwise clinically silent presentation.

AUDIOGRAM

A formal audiogram is advised in all patients reporting persistent or sudden hearing loss and in any patient with new otologic symptoms and a prior history of ear surgery or chronic ear disease. The audiogram is an extremely valuable diagnostic tool. In addition to categorizing the type of hearing loss, assessing brainstem reflexes, and evaluating the compliance of the tympanic membrane, information attained from a complete audiometric evaluation may provide critical context to guide management decisions.

Laboratory Studies

Serologic studies in the workup of otalgia are not routinely recommended. However, they maybe diagnostically beneficial or required in certain clinical situations. If severe infection is involved, the patient should be assessed for serologic markers of infection, including complete blood count, erythrocyte sedimentation rate, and C-reactive protein. For patients who are under consideration for autoimmune disease, a full autoimmune panel is not required for isolated otalgia without hearing loss or other symptoms, and targeted serologic studies should be pursued. If the patient also reports fluctuating hearing loss, progressive hearing loss, or episodic vertigo in a Meniere-like syndrome, referral to otolaryngology is recommended for further evaluation. Based on the results of that assessment, the patient may require a full complement of serologic studies to thoroughly evaluate for systemic manifestations of otologic disease.

With respect to other laboratory studies, routine culture data are not necessary in uncomplicated and nonrecurrent otitis externa or otitis media. However, patients with apparent treatment-refractory disease should undergo culture swab for speciation and sensitivity analysis. As previously noted, referral to an otolaryngologist is recommended for clinic-based biopsy when granulation tissue is identified in the external auditory canal to rule out malignancy as an underlying cause, even when malignant otitis externa is the expected diagnosis.

Radiographic Studies

Imaging is not indicated in the general diagnostic workup of otalgia but may be advisable in the right clinical scenario. Patients with suspicion for intratemporal complications of otologic infectious disease (eg, mastoiditis) may benefit from CT with thin cuts of the temporal bone in anticipation of possible surgical intervention. Those who are suspected to have an occult malignancy, particularly with examination abnormalities affecting the parapharyngeal space, may undergo an MRI of the orbit/face/neck with and without gadolinium in addition to CT. Any patients with a suspected intracranial complication of infectious disease or focal neurologic deficits should undergo MRI brain with and without contrast.

Consultation and Referrals

As discussed throughout this article, otalgia has an underlying differential diagnosis that encompasses multiple organ systems across multiple medical disciplines. Most patients have a diagnostically apparent cause, most commonly ear infection, TMJ disorder, or dental pathology. However, a significant portion of patients do not fall into one of these categories. As a result, the patient's journey to resolution may not be linear, and the evaluation of their complaints may often require multidisciplinary coordination. In addition to primary care, emergency medicine, and otolaryngology, numerous specialties may assist in the evaluation of otalgia, including oral surgery/general dentistry, dermatology, rheumatology, neurology, neurosurgery, infectious disease, and gastroenterology, among others. In some rare cases, no specific cause is found, and pain medicine contributes in the management of the patient's bothersome symptoms. Thorough initial evaluation and workup of their symptoms may yield critical insights with respect to which specialty is most likely to offer the patient diagnostic insight and therapeutic benefit.

SUMMARY

Otalgia is a bothersome symptom leading to a significant number of outpatient and emergency department visits annually. Because of the numerous potential causes and primary sources of otalgia, a systematic approach to evaluation is critical to properly evaluate and elucidate a diagnosis that will ultimately guide symptom relief. The presence of hearing loss and/or otorrhea highly suggests primary otologic disease, but isolated otalgia is nearly always resultant of disease processes external to the ear. Providers should retain a global understanding of the underlying anatomic rationale for referred ear pain and avoid overdiagnosis and treatment of "ear infection" in patients with isolated otalgia. In some cases, a multidisciplinary approach will be essential to accurate diagnosis and effective management. Although a preponderance of isolated otalgia is attributable to TMJ disorder or dental pathology, severe unilateral otalgia may portend a more ominous diagnosis, such as an occult malignancy. Clinicians should have a low threshold for further evaluation of persistent unilateral otalgia that is unresponsive to conservative management, particularly in the presence of risk factor for malignancy or alarm symptoms.

CLINICS CARE POINTS

- Otalgia can be broadly categorized as primary otalgia (arising from disorders of auricle and ear) and secondary otalgia (also known as nonotogenic; arising from disorders other than the ear).
- The ear has a robust nerve supply involving 5 cranial and cervical nerves, which can cause otalgia in a wide variety of conditions due to referred pain.
- Primary otalgia is nearly always associated with concurrent audiovestibular symptoms such as hearing loss, vertigo, or otorrhea.
- Isolated otalgia without hearing loss, otorrhea, or abnormal otoscopic findings is most commonly referred pain, and the most common cause is the TMJ disorder.
- Persistent, progressive unilateral otalgia or a unilateral middle ear effusion warrants evaluation for a nasopharyngeal mass with nasal endoscopy and/or further imaging.
- Alarm symptoms such as progressive facial palsy, severe pain, or other cranial neuropathy warrant evaluation with further imaging.

DISCLOSURE

The authors have nothing to disclose.

REFERENCES

1. Kozin ED, Sethi RK, Remenschneider AK, et al. Epidemiology of otologic diagnoses in U nited S tates emergency departments. Laryngoscope 2015;125(8):1926–33.
2. Kim SH, Kim TH, Byun JY, et al. Clinical differences in types of otalgia. J Audiol Otol 2015;19(1):34.
3. Cummings C. Cummings otolaryngology head & neck surgery. Philadelphia: Elselver Mosby; 2005.
4. Dalal PJ, Purkey MR, Price CP, et al. Risk factors for auricular hematoma and recurrence after drainage. Laryngoscope 2020;130(3):628–31.
5. Giles WC, Iverson KC, King JD, et al. Incision and drainage followed by mattress suture repair of auricular hematoma. Laryngoscope 2007;117(12):2097–9.
6. Bassiouny A. Perichondritis of the auricle. Laryngoscope 1981;91(3):422–31.
7. Kechichian E, Jabbour S, Haber R, et al. Management of chondrodermatitis nodularis helicis: a systematic review and treatment algorithm. Dermatol Surg 2016; 42(10):1125–34.
8. Roland PS, Stroman DW. Microbiology of acute otitis externa. Laryngoscope 2002;112(7):1166–77.
9. Coulson S, Croxson GR, Adams R, et al. Prognostic factors in herpes zoster oticus (Ramsay Hunt syndrome). Otol Neurotol 2011;32(6):1025–30.
10. Uscategui T, Doree C, Chamberlain IJ, et al. Corticosteroids as adjuvant to antiviral treatment in Ramsay Hunt syndrome (herpes zoster oticus with facial palsy) in adults. Cochrane Database Syst Rev 2008;(3):CD006852.
11. Kansu L, Yilmaz I. Herpes zoster oticus (Ramsay Hunt syndrome) in children: case report and literature review. Int J Pediatr Otorhinolaryngol 2012;76(6):772–6.
12. Sylvester MJ, Sanghvi S, Patel VM, et al. Malignant otitis externa hospitalizations: analysis of patient characteristics. Laryngoscope 2017;127(10):2328–36.
13. Sturm JJ, Stern Shavit S, Lalwani AK. What is the best test for diagnosing and monitoring treatment response in malignant otitis media? The Laryngoscope 2020;130(11):2516–7.

14. Prasad N, Harley E. The aural foreign body space: A review of pediatric ear foreign bodies and a management paradigm. Int J Pediatr Otorhinolaryngol 2020;132:109871.

15. Goff CJ, Allred C, Glade RS. Current management of congenital branchial cleft cysts, sinuses, and fistulae. Curr Opin Otolaryngol Head Neck Surg 2012; 20(6):533–9.

16. Sharon JD, Khwaja SS, Drescher A, et al. Osteoradionecrosis of the temporal bone: a case series. Otol Neurotol 2014;35(7):1207.

17. Lou ZC, Lou ZH, Zhang QP. Traumatic tympanic membrane perforations: a study of etiology and factors affecting outcome. Am J Otolaryngol 2012;33(5):549–55.

18. Lieberthal AS, Carroll AE, Chonmaitree T, Ganiats TG, Hoberman A, Jackson MA,, Schwartz RH. The diagnosis and management of acute otitis media. Pediatrics 2013;131(3):e964–99.

19. Limb CJ, Lustig LR, Klein JO. Acute otitis media in adults. Welthem, MA: UpToDate; 2018.

20. Yorgancılar E, Yıldırım M, Gun R, et al. Complications of chronic suppurative otitis media: a retrospective review. Eur Arch Otorhinolaryngol 2013;270(1):69–76.

21. Kaya S, Tsuprun V, Hızlı Ö, et al. Quantitative assessment of cochlear histopathologic findings in patients with suppurative labyrinthitis. JAMA Otolaryngol Head Neck Surg 2016;142(4):364–9.

22. Gadre AK, Chole RA. The changing face of petrous apicitis—a 40-year experience. Laryngoscope 2018;128(1):195–201.

23. Ely JW, Hansen MR, Clark EC. Diagnosis of ear pain. Am Fam Physician 2008; 77(5):621–8.

24. Kuttila SJ, Kuttila MH, Niemi PM, et al. Secondary otalgia in an adult population. Arch Otolaryngol Head Neck Surg 2001;127(4):401–5.

25. Visvanathan V, Kelly G. 12 minute consultation: an evidence-based management of referred otalgia. Clin Otolaryngol 2010;35(5):409–14.

26. Scarbrough TJ, Day TA, Williams TE, et al. Referred otalgia in head and neck cancer: a unifying schema. Am J Clin Oncol 2003;26(5):e157–62.

27. Jaber JJ, Leonetti JP, Lawrason AE, et al. Cervical spine causes for referred otalgia. Otolaryngol Head Neck Surg 2008;138(4):479–85.

28. Beder E, Ozgursoy OB, Ozgursoy SK, et al. Three-dimensional computed tomography and surgical treatment for Eagle's syndrome. Ear Nose Throat J 2006;85(7): 443–5.

29. Piagkou M, Anagnostopoulou S, Kouladouros K, et al. Eagle's syndrome: a review of the literature. Clin Anat 2009;22(5):545–58.

30. Teixido M, Seymour P, Kung B, et al. Otalgia associated with migraine. Otol Neurotol 2011;32(2):322–5.

31. Birnbaum J. Facial weakness, otalgia, and hemifacial spasm: a novel neurological syndrome in a case-series of 3 patients with rheumatic disease. Medicine 2015;94(40):e1445.

32. Suneja A, Madani S. Neuropathic Otalgia: Rare and Treatable Ear Pains. Neurology 2020;94 (15 Supplement) 2583.

33. Olds MJ, Woods CI, Winfield JA. Microvascular decompression in glossopharyngeal neuralgia. Otol Neurotol 1995;16(3):326–30.

34. Earwood JS, Rogers T, Rathjen NA. Ear pain: diagnosing common and uncommon causes. Am Fam Physician 2018;97(1):20–7.

35. Takagi D, Nakamaru Y, Maguchi S, et al. Otologic manifestations of Wegener's granulomatosis. Laryngoscope 2002;112(9):1684–90.

36. Shah UK, White JA, Gooey JE, et al. Otolaryngologic manifestations of sarcoidosis: presentation and diagnosis. Laryngoscope 1997;107(1):67–75.

37. Gaudet JE, Walvekar RR, Arriaga MA, et al. Applicability of the Pittsburgh staging system for advanced cutaneous malignancy of the temporal bone. Skull Base 2010;20(6):409.

38. Hill BA, Kohut RI. Metastatic adenocarcinoma of the temporal bone. Arch Otolaryngol 1976;102(9):568–71.

39. Lan MY, Shiao AS, Li WY. Facial paralysis caused by metastasis of breast carcinoma to the temporal bone. J Chin Med Assoc 2004;67(11):587–90.

Evaluation and Management of a Neck Mass

Kevin Chorath, MD[a], Karthik Rajasekaran, MD[a,b,*]

KEYWORDS

- Neck mass • Neck cancer • Evaluation of neck • Neck lesion
- Head and neck cancer

KEY POINTS

- There are several reasons for patients to present with neck masses, but the most important etiology to rule out is malignancy.
- Antibiotics may be provided if the patient has an exam consistent with bacterial infection. However, further evaluation is necessary if the mass persists or reoccurs.
- The initial imaging test of choice to evaluate a persistent or recurring neck mass is a CT or MRI scan with intravenous contrast.
- Fine needle aspiration (FNA) is the initial test of choice for biopsying a concerning neck mass.
- Inconclusive testing results for a cystic or persistent neck mass warrants repeat workup and referrals to specialists.

INTRODUCTION

Patients presenting with neck masses are a common occurrence. Neck masses are abnormal lesions that are located below the mandible, above the clavicle, and deep to the skin. They can be visible, palpable, or seen on imaging studies. Discerning the underlying pathology of these masses is often not easy and can be quite challenging. Neck masses may develop from infectious, inflammatory, congenital, traumatic, benign, or malignant processes.[1,2] Unlike in children in whom the most common cause for a neck mass is infection, adults neck masses are most commonly caused by malignancy. In fact, there is ample literature to suggest that a persistent neck mass in an adult patient should be considered malignant until proved otherwise.[2,3] As such, further investigation is paramount in adults because it may be the only manifestation of malignancy of the head and neck. The location of the mass, imaging findings, and relevant historical information are important considerations when differentiating various causes of neck masses.[1,2,4–6] The goal of this article is to

[a] Department of Otorhinolaryngology–Head and Neck Surgery, University of Pennsylvania, Philadelphia, PA, USA; [b] Leonard Davis Institute of Health Economics, University of Pennsylvania, Philadelphia, PA, USA
* Corresponding author. 800 Walnut Street, 18th Floor, Philadelphia, PA 19107.
E-mail address: Karthik.Rajasekaran@pennmedicine.upenn.edu

Med Clin N Am 105 (2021) 827–837
https://doi.org/10.1016/j.mcna.2021.05.005
0025-7125/21/© 2021 Elsevier Inc. All rights reserved.

medical.theclinics.com

provide a working framework to understand, diagnose, and manage neck masses that present in the outpatient setting.

HISTORY

A thorough medical history can provide important information to the diagnosis of a neck mass. Key details to ascertain include the following:

- *Age:* the age of the patient provides important information about possible causes of the mass. It is one of the most significant predictors of malignancy.[5]
- *Characteristics of the mass:* information related to the duration, growth pattern, and presence of pain can provide clues about the cause of the mass.
- *Associated symptoms:* the presence of hoarseness, stridor, dysphagia, odynophagia, otalgia, and epistaxis suggests cervical metastasis from a primary malignancy of the upper aerodigestive tract.[6] Providers should also ask about systemic symptoms and classic "B signs" of lymphoma, including fever, chills, night sweats, and unintentional weight loss.
- *Social history:* this includes tobacco use (amount, duration, and method), alcohol use, intravenous drug use, animal contact, and recent travel.

PHYSICAL EXAMINATION

A thorough head and neck examination can provide additional details about the cause of the mass. Key components include

- *Characteristics of mass*
  - Size
  - Location
  - Quality (soft, fluctuant, rubbery, firm)
  - Mobility (mobile, hypomobile, or immobile)
  - Tenderness
  - Skin changes (erythema of overlying skin, fixed to skin)
- Head and neck examination
  - Skin—evaluate the face and scalp for lesions, ulcerations, erythema
  - Oral cavity and oropharynx—examine the tonsil, palate, posterior pharynx, tongue, tongue mobility, buccal mucosa, and gingiva. Dentures or other dental appliances should ideally be removed. Note any erythema, ulcerations, diminished movements, or asymmetry. Palpation of these structures can reveal occult lesions.
  - Nose—examine the external nose, nasal mucosa, septum, and turbinates and assess for sinus tenderness
  - Ear—assess for diminished hearing and effusions with otoscopic examination
  - Larynx—palpation during swallowing as well as assessing for laryngeal crepitus may reveal underlying pathology
  - Cranial nerves

IMAGING

Imaging should be ordered for patients with a neck mass deemed at increased risk for malignancy. The 2 main imaging modalities that are recommended are contrast-enhanced computed tomography (CT) or MRI scans:

- *CT scan:* CT scan represents the most widely used imaging modality for the head and neck region and is the initial diagnostic test of choice for patients with a persistent neck mass.[7] There are several advantages to a CT scan, including wide-spread availability, quick acquisition, and low cost. It is an excellent initial imaging test because of its ability to characterize the mass in relation to other structures in the head and neck and assess involvement of deep neck spaces. Although CT uses ionizing radiation, it is considered acceptable in the adult population.[8]

- *MRI:* similar to the CT scan, MRI allows for precise localization of the mass and can accurately characterize tumors and inflammation. Although both studies are effective for oncologic evaluation, MRI provides superior visualization of soft-tissue and possible perineural extension.[9] The advantages of MRI include lack of radiation exposure, and the image quality is preserved in patients with dental restorations such as crowns, caps, or implants.[10] However, MRIs are costlier, challenging for patients with claustrophobia, take longer (~30 minutes), and are precluded in patients with certain implantable medical devices such as pacemakers.

Irrespective of which imaging modality is selected, the addition of intravenous contrast is essential unless there is a contraindication, such as contrast allergy or renal insufficiency.[11] There is rarely any added benefit for ordering a scan without contrast and therefore should be avoided. Contrast improves characterization of the mass, maps out the borders, and can better identify the relationship of the neck mass to major vessels.

The other imaging modality often used is an ultrasound (US). US represents the least invasive imaging techniques and can provide real-time assessment of the mass and image-guided sampling. US can adequately characterize benign, vascular, inflammatory, and malignant lesions and is the gold standard for evaluating the thyroid.[12] However, there are several disadvantages when using this tool. US is limited for its evaluation of deep spaces of the neck and is highly operator-dependent.[13] It is therefore not recommended as a first option. The few exceptions to this are if there is a delay in obtaining CT/MRI, the use of contrast is contraindicated, or it is needed as an adjunct to expedite a fine-needle aspiration biopsy (FNA).[14]

BIOPSY

When the diagnosis of a neck mass remains uncertain, a biopsy should be performed. FNA represents the gold standard should be the initial test for histologic evaluation.[15] FNA is a procedure by which a small caliber needle, typically a 25- or 27-gauge needle, is inserted into the mass to obtain a small sample.[16] FNA can be done without preoperative clearance and does not expose patients to the risks of anesthesia. They can be performed with and without image guidance using a US or CT scan. It is highly accurate, safe, cost-effective, and provides timely diagnosis and less morbidity compared with an open biopsy.

Although FNA of neck masses is highly accurate, some results may not provide a definitive answer; this can occur because there is insufficient amount of lesional material for the pathologist to make a diagnosis, which is usually described as an inadequate specimen.[17] The other reason why this may occur is when there is adequate specimen but the cells obtained in the sample do not provide a specific diagnosis. In both scenarios, if the patient has worrisome signs and symptoms for a malignancy or has a persistent neck mass, a repeat FNA should be attempted before resorting to an open biopsy.[3]

If the results of the FNA are inadequate or indeterminate to provide a diagnosis, a core needle biopsy may be considered. Core needle is typically performed under local anesthesia and uses a larger gauge needle compared with FNA (~14–18 gauge) for tissue extraction. Core needle biopsies may also be preferred in settings of suspected cases of lymphoma, as it allows for greater appreciation of tissue architecture.[18] However, core needle biopsies do increase the chance for trauma from using larger-bore needles, as well as increase the risk for tumor seeding, the latter being the reason why it is contraindicated in patients with concerns for a squamous cell carcinoma.[19]

An open biopsy, on the other hand, is the most definitive way of obtaining a diagnosis. It involves making an incision on the neck and removing the entire mass or a portion of the mass[20]; this is typically done under local anesthesia at minimum and often performed in an operating room. Because it is more invasive than an FNA, it should be reserved for those scenarios that an FNA has failed to provide a diagnosis or more tissue is required by the pathologists.[21]

ANCILLARY TESTING

Certain laboratory tests may be useful and can be ordered based on clinical suspicion for a specific disease.[22] **Box 1** highlights some of the laboratory tests that may be considered.

DIFFERENTIAL DIAGNOSIS

The common causes of a neck mass in adult can be classified into 6 major categories:

- Congenital
  - Thyroglossal duct cyst: this represents the most common congenital anomaly of the head and neck region, and although most commonly seen in children, remnants can be present in 7% of the adult population.[23] These malformations can develop anywhere between the base of tongue down to the thyroid's native position in the neck. Most commonly, they present as midline cysts near the hyoid bone that elevate with protrusion of the tongue or swallowing.[24] These masses can be observed or surgically removed via a Sistrunk procedure, which involves removal of the cyst along with a portion of the hyoid bone.[25]

Box 1
Laboratory tests for evaluation of neck mass

Complete blood count (CBC) with differential

Erythrocyte semination rate (ESR) and C-reactive protein (CRP)

Serology for Epstein-Barr virus (EBV) or cytomegalovirus (CMV)

Serology for human immunodeficiency virus (HIV)

Antineutrophil antibody (ANA)

Thyroid stimulating hormone (TSH) and free T4

Parathyroid hormone (PTH)

Serology for toxoplasma, brucellosis, bartonella, tularemia

Tuberculin skin test

Antibodies to Ro/SSA and La/SSB

- Branchial cleft cyst: this congenital anomaly can arise from any of the first through fourth pharyngeal clefts.[26] Similar to the thyroglossal duct cyst, they are usually present at birth but become obvious or symptomatic in childhood. Rarely, these cysts can persist into adulthood and are often discovered when they become tender, enlarged, or inflamed after an upper respiratory infection. They can also become infected and lead to purulent drainage to the external skin or pharynx.[27] Treatment entails surgical excision.
- Venolymphatic malformations
  - Cystic hygroma (lymphangioma): this represents a benign congenital anomaly of the lymphatic system most commonly presenting in children, but seldom presents *de novo* in adult patients.[28] These lymphatic malformations can present anywhere in the head and neck region as a painless, soft, fluctuant, enlarging neck mass. The cause is unknown but likely due to acquired processes such as infection, surgical manipulation, or lymphatic obstruction.[29] These masses can be observed or treated via sclerotherapy or surgery.[30]
  - Hemangiomas: these vascular malformations are typically present at birth and rapidly proliferate in the first few years of childhood but eventually involute.[31] Sometimes, patients may have residual telangiectasias, scarring, or atrophy, which presents as a mass and may need treatment. Several treatment options exist, including laser therapy, sclerotherapy, or surgery.[32]
  - Venous malformations: these arise from abnormal, ectatic venous channels and often present in the head and neck region. Similar to hemangiomas, venous malformations can be present at birth; however, they tend to grow as the patient ages without spontaneous resolution.[33] Depending on their size, architecture, location, and flow rate, they can be asymptomatic or can cause significant morbidity including pain, discomfort, life-threatening bleeding, or respiratory compromise. Current treatment strategies include surgery, laser therapy, or sclerotherapy.[34]
  - Pseudoaneurysm or arteriovenous fistula: these may occur as a result of shearing or penetrating trauma to the neck and present as a soft, pulsatile mass with a thrill or bruit.[35] These masses are potentially lethal and require prompt treatment to prevent rupture or neurologic dysfunction. Standard treatment in the past entailed surgical repair and ligation of the carotid artery. However, more recently, endovascular techniques with stent grafts have evolved as effective options.[36]
- Infectious
  - Viral infection: there are a variety of viral agents that can cause cervical lymphadenopathy. The most common viral pathogens causing upper respiratory infection include rhinovirus, coronavirus, and influenza and resulting lymphadenopathy typically subsides within 3 to 6 weeks after symptom resolution.[37]
  - Bartonella henselae: this is the etiologic agent of cat-scratch disease, and classically, these patients present after a bite/scratch by an infected cat.[38] Patients can develop a bulbous or vesicular lesion at site of inoculation, followed by ipsilateral lymphadenopathy in the cervical, inguinal, or axillary region. Treatment typically entails a 5-day course of azithromycin.[39]
  - Tuberculous cervical lymphadenitis: tuberculosis (TB) of the lymph nodes is one of the most common extrapulmonary manifestation of the disease.[40] It can be caused by tuberculous or nontuberculous mycobacterium and can be seen in immunocompromised patients or in patients with recent travel to endemic regions. It usually presents as a chronic, painless neck mass without

apparent signs of infection such as warmth or edema.[41] This finding may be accompanied by other constitutional signs of TB, including night sweats, chills, and unintentional weight loss.

- Benign neoplasm
  - Lipoma: these are benign, subcutaneous masses of mesenchymal origin that can present in the head and neck region.[42] These tumors are usually smooth and mobile and are often asymptomatic. These masses can be observed or surgically excised.
  - Thyroid nodule: thyroid nodules are common and can be seen in 65% of the population.[43] Most thyroid nodules are benign and incidentally found on imaging. The gold standard for evaluating a thyroid nodule is an ultrasound. The results of the ultrasound are typically reported as a Thyroid Imaging Reporting & Data System (TI-RADS) score.[43] Management of the thyroid nodule depends on the size of the nodule in combination with the TI-RADS score, which can either be observation or an FNA of the nodule.[14] The results of an FNA are typically reported using the Bethesda Classification,[44] the results of which and subsequent management are outside the scope of this article and therefore not discussed.
- Malignant Neoplasm
  - Malignancy of upper aerodigestive tract: malignancies in the oral cavity, nasopharynx, oropharynx, sinonasal cavity, hypopharynx, and larynx can metastasize to the neck presenting as a neck mass.[3] The most common malignancy is squamous cell carcinoma (SCC), which is typically caused by alcohol, smoking, and more recently the human papilloma virus (HPV).[45] The presentation of patients with SCC in the head and neck caused by smoking and alcohol is quite different than those caused by HPV. SCC caused by smoking and alcohol typically present with neck painful masses in the upper aerodigestive tract, along with other symptoms including dysphagia, odynophagia, change in voice, or ear pain. On the other hand, patients with SCC caused by HPV typically present with only a painless neck mass. Most of them have no other symptoms and are often misdiagnosed as having a branchial cleft cyst.[46] Management of upper aerodigestive tract cancers depends on the location and stage of the cancer.[47]
  - Thyroid cancer: the most common type of thyroid cancer is papillary. Other cancers of the thyroid gland include follicular, medullary, and anaplastic.[48] Generally, thyroid cancer has a very good prognosis, with the exception being anaplastic thyroid carcinoma. Management of thyroid cancer typically involves a thyroidectomy and can include adjuvant radioactive iodine based on the pathology.[43]
  - Salivary gland cancer: salivary gland cancers can originate from major (parotid, submandibular, and sublingual) or minor (located throughout the upper aerodigestive tract) salivary glands. Management of these cancers typically involves surgery followed by adjuvant therapy based on pathology.
  - Lymphoma: cervical lymphadenopathy is one of the most common manifestations of lymphoma. Lymphoma can generally be classified as Hodgkin lymphoma (HL) and non-Hodgkin lymphoma (NHL).[49] HL typically involves lymph nodes in the neck, whereas NHL can spread to extranodal sites, including the major salivary glands, paranasal sinuses, and Waldeyer ring.[50] Imaging findings are incapable of differentiating these 2 forms. Management typically involves chemotherapy and sometimes addition of radiation therapy.[51]

- ○ Metastasis of thoracoabdominal malignancy: occasionally, malignancies from the abdomen and thorax can metastasize to a supraclavicular node, known as Virchow node.[52] Management of these cancers is based on the underlying malignancy.
- Systemic diseases
  - ○ Sjogren syndrome: this is an autoimmune disease that commonly presents in older women. Patients typically present with dry eyes and mouth and many

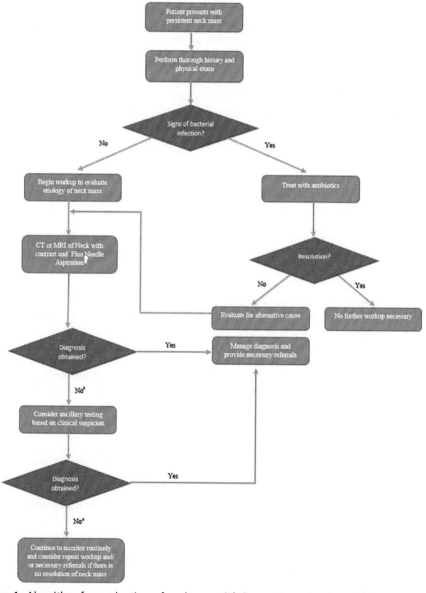

Fig. 1. Algorithm for evaluation of neck mass. [a]If diagnostic evaluation yields cystic neck mass, further testing is necessary to rule out malignancy.

also exhibit persistent enlargement of the submandibular or parotid gland. Patients may have elevated levels of antineutrophil antibody and rheumatoid factor, as well as antibodies to anti-Ro/SS-A or anti-La/SSB; however, these antibodies are not specific to Sjogren syndrome and can be seen in other autoimmune diseases. Treatment is focused on managing the symptoms, including topical tear replacement for xerophthalmia and oral hygiene to increase salivary flow.

o Sarcoidosis: this inflammatory syndrome is characterized by the development of granulomas, leading to permanent scarring or thickening of organ tissue.[53] Signs and symptoms depend on the location of the granulomas, and up to 10% to 15% of patients can exhibit head and neck manifestations.[54] In many cases, sarcoidosis will resolve on its own; however, several therapies including steroids, immunosuppressants, and antimalarial medication can control symptom and prevent further destruction.[55]

o Other autoimmune disease: several conditions including rheumatoid arthritis, systemic lupus erythematosus, scleroderma, and vasculitis can have manifestations in the head and neck region and may be the sole presenting feature.[56] Laboratory testing is needed to classify the specific type of autoimmune disease, and management is dictated by the type of the disease.[57]

MANAGEMENT

The management of a neck mass depends on the underlying cause. **Fig. 1** provides an algorithm to guide the management of these patients. Because the most common cause for a neck mass is infection, it is reasonable to prescribe a course of antibiotics and reevaluate in 2 weeks for resolution. Patients who do not respond appropriately or have a recurrence of the neck mass warrant further evaluation.

SUMMARY

There are several causes of neck masses, and discerning an accurate cause can be challenging. Using a systematic approach will usually result in an accurate diagnosis and guide appropriate treatment. A careful medical history and physical examination can provide important clues as to the diagnosis and dictate the need for follow-up evaluation with imaging, tissue biopsies, and necessary referrals. The most important cause that must be ruled out is malignancy. In cases where a diagnosis is not obtained, patients should be monitored closely. If the mass fails to resolve or recurs, repeat workup and/or specialist referrals should be considered.

CLINICS CARE POINTS

- There are several reasons for patients to present with neck masses, but the most important cause to rule out is malignancy.

- Antibiotics may be provided if the patient has a history and physical examination consistent with a bacterial infection. However, further evaluation is necessary if the mass persists or reoccurs.

- The initial imaging test of choice to evaluate a persistent or recurring neck mass is a CT or MRI scan with intravenous contrast.

- FNA is the initial test of choice for biopsying a concerning neck mass.

- Inconclusive testing results for a cystic or persistent neck mass warrant repeat workup and referrals to specialists.

DISCLOSURE

The authors have nothing to disclose.

REFERENCES

1. Olsen KD. Evaluation of masses in the neck. Prim Care 1990;17(2):415–35. Available at: https://pubmed.ncbi.nlm.nih.gov/2196618/. Accessed November 30, 2020.
2. Rosenberg TL, Brown JJ, Jefferson GD. Evaluating the adult patient with a neck mass. Med Clin North Am 2010;94(5):1017–29.
3. Pynnonen MA, Gillespie MB, Roman B, et al. Clinical Practice Guideline: Evaluation of the Neck Mass in Adults. Otolaryngol Head Neck Surg 2017;157(2_suppl):S1–30.
4. Lefebvre JL, Coche-Dequeant B, Ton Van J, et al. Cervical lymph nodes from an unknown primary tumor in 190 patients. Am J Surg 1990;160(4):443–6.
5. Bhattacharyya N. Predictive factors for neoplasia and malignancy in a neck mass. Arch Otolaryngol Head Neck Surg 1999;125(3):303–7.
6. Haynes J, Arnold KR, Aguirre-Oskins C, et al. Evaluation of Neck Masses in Adults. Vol 91. 2015. Available at: www.aafp.org/afp. Accessed November 30, 2020.
7. Wippold FJ. Head and neck imaging: The role of CT and MRI. J Magn Reson Imaging 2007;25(3):453–65.
8. Colagrande S, Origgi D, Zatelli G, et al. CT exposure in adult and paediatric patients: A review of the mechanisms of damage, relative dose and consequent possible risks. Radiol Med 2014;119(10):803–10.
9. Dammann F, Bootz F, Cohnen M, et al. Bildgebende verfahren in der kopf-hals-diagnostik. Dtsch Arztebl Int 2014;111(23–24):417–23.
10. Supsupin EP, Demian NM. Magnetic Resonance Imaging (MRI) in the diagnosis of head and neck disease. Oral Maxillofac Surg Clin North Am 2014;26(2):253–69.
11. Chow GV, Nazarian S. MRI for patients with cardiac implantable electrical devices. Cardiol Clin 2014;32(2):299–304.
12. Novoa E, Gürtler N, Arnoux A, et al. Role of ultrasound-guided core-needle biopsy in the assessment of head and neck lesions: A meta-analysis and systematic review of the literature. Head Neck 2012;34(10):1497–503.
13. Alberico RA, Husain SHS, Sirotkin I. Imaging in head and neck oncology. Surg Oncol Clin N Am 2004;13(1):13–35.
14. Nabhan F, Ringel MD. Thyroid nodules and cancer management guidelines: Comparisons and controversies. Endocr Relat Cancer 2017;24(2):R13–26.
15. Learned KO, Lev-Toaff AS, Brake BJ, et al. US-guided biopsy of neck lesions: The head and neck neuroradiologist's perspective. Radiographics 2016;36(1):226–43.
16. Layfield LJ. Fine-needle aspiration in the diagnosis of head and neck lesions: A review and discussion of problems in differential diagnosis. Diagn Cytopathol 2007;35:798–805.
17. Amedee RG, Dhurandhar NR. Fine-needle aspiration biopsy. Laryngoscope 2001;111(9):1551–7.
18. Jiang ST, Smith RV. Is core needle biopsy safe and effective for the assessment of head and neck lesions? Laryngoscope 2018;128(12):2669–70.
19. Cho J, Kim J, Lee JS, et al. Comparison of core needle biopsy and fine-needle aspiration in diagnosis of ma lignant salivary gland neoplasm: Systematic review and meta-analysis. Head Neck 2020;42(10):3041–50.

20. Adoga AA, Silas OA, Nimkur TL. Open cervical lymph node biopsy for head and neck cancers: any benefit? Head Neck Oncol 2009;1:9.

21. Akkina SR, Kim RY, Stucken CL, et al. The current practice of open neck mass biopsy in the diagnosis of head and neck cancer: A retrospective cohort study. Laryngoscope Investig Otolaryngol 2019;4(1):57–61.

22. Evaluation of a neck mass in adults - UpToDate. Available at: https://www.uptodate.com/contents/evaluation-of-a-neck-mass-in-adults. Accessed December 1, 2020.

23. Carter Y, Yeutter N, Mazeh H. Thyroglossal duct remnant carcinoma: beyond the Sistrunk procedure. Surg Oncol 2014;23(3):161–6.

24. Agnoni AA. Thyroglossal duct cyst. In: Coppola C, Kennedy Jr. A, Scorpio R, editors. Pediatric surgery: diagnosis and treatment. Cham: Springer International Publishing; 2014. p. 237–40. https://doi.org/10.1007/978-3-319-04340-1_41.

25. Gallagher TQ, Hartnick CJ. Thyroglossal duct cyst excision. Adv Otorhinolaryngol 2012;73:66–9.

26. Branchial Cleft Cyst - StatPearls - NCBI Bookshelf. Available at: https://www.ncbi.nlm.nih.gov/books/NBK499914/. Accessed December 1, 2020.

27. Makowski AL. Second branchial cleft cyst. J Emerg Med 2014;47(1):76–7.

28. Dogruyol T, Tozum H, Eren TS. Rapidly growing cystic hygroma in an adult patient. Asian Cardiovasc Thorac Ann 2017;25(5):395–7.

29. Carretero RG, Rodriguez-Maya B, Vazquez-Gomez O. Non-surgical treatment of a relapsed cystic hygroma in an adult. BMJ Case Rep 2017;2017. https://doi.org/10.1136/bcr-2016-218783.

30. Ha J, Yu Y-C, Lannigan F. A Review of the Management of Lymphangiomas. Curr Pediatr Rev 2017;10(3):238–48.

31. JACOBS AH. Strawberry hemangiomas; the natural history of the untreated lesion. Calif Med 1957;86(1):8–10.

32. Satterfield KR, Chambers CB. Current treatment and management of infantile hemangiomas. Surv Ophthalmol 2019;64(5):608–18.

33. Park H, Kim JS, Park H, et al. Venous malformations of the head and neck: A retrospective review of 82 cases. Arch Plast Surg 2019;46(1):23–33.

34. Zheng JW, Mai HM, Zhang L, et al. Guidelines for the treatment of head and neck venous malformations. Int J Clin Exp Med 2013;6(5):377–89. Available at: www.ijcem.com/. Accessed December 1, 2020.

35. Youssef AS, Downes AE. Intraoperative neurophysiological monitoring in vestibular schwannoma surgery: Advances and clinical implications. Neurosurg Focus 2009;27(4):E9.

36. Cox MW, Whittaker DR, Martinez C, et al. Traumatic pseudoaneurysms of the head and neck: Early endovascular intervention. J Vasc Surg 2007;46(6):1227–33.

37. Leung AK, Robson WLM. Childhood cervical lymphadenopathy. J Pediatr Heal Care 2004;18(1):3–7.

38. Microbiology, epidemiology, clinical manifestations, and diagnosis of cat scratch disease - UpToDate. Available at: https://www.uptodate.com/contents/microbiology-epidemiology-clinical-manifestations-and-diagnosis-of-cat-scratch-disease. Accessed December 1, 2020.

39. Treatment of cat scratch disease - UpToDate. Available at: https://www.uptodate.com/contents/treatment-of-cat-scratch-disease#H4276501801. Accessed December 1, 2020.

40. Haynes J, Arnold KR, Aguirre-Oskins C, et al. Evaluation of neck masses in adults. Am Fam Physician 2015;91(10):698–706.

41. Hegde S, Rithesh KB, Baroudi K, et al. Tuberculous lymphadenitis: early diagnosis and intervention. J Int Oral Heal 2014;6(6):96–8. Available at: http://www.ncbi.nlm.nih.gov/pubmed/25628495. Accessed December 1, 2020.

42. Kolb L, Yarrarapu SNS, Ameer MA, et al. Lipoma. Florida: StatPearls Publishing; 2020. Available at: http://www.ncbi.nlm.nih.gov/pubmed/29939683. Accessed December 1, 2020.

43. Haugen BR. 2015 American Thyroid Association Management Guidelines for Adult Patients with Thyroid Nodules and Differentiated Thyroid Cancer: What is new and what has changed? Cancer 2017;123(3):372–81.

44. Cibas ES, Ali SZ. The 2017 Bethesda System for Reporting Thyroid Cytopathology. Thyroid 2017;27(11):1341–6.

45. Chow LQM. Head and Neck Cancer. N Engl J Med 2020;382(1):60–72.

46. Syrjänen S, Rautava J, Syrjänen K. HPV in head and neck cancer—30 years of history. Recent Results Cancer Res 2017;206:3–25.

47. Huang SH, O'Sullivan B. Overview of the 8th Edition TNM Classification for Head and Neck Cancer. Curr Treat Options Oncol 2017;18(7).

48. Cabanillas ME, McFadden DG, Durante C. Thyroid cancer. Lancet 2016; 388(10061):2783–95.

49. Armitage JO, Gascoyne RD, Lunning MA, et al. Non-Hodgkin lymphoma. Lancet 2017;390(10091):298–310.

50. Kaseb H, Babiker HM. Cancer, lymphoma, Hodgkin. Florida: StatPearls Publishing; 2018. Available at: http://www.ncbi.nlm.nih.gov/pubmed/29763144. Accessed December 1, 2020.

51. Matasar MJ, Zelenetz AD. Overview of Lymphoma Diagnosis and Management. Radiol Clin North Am 2008;46(2):175–98.

52. Zdilla MJ, Aldawood AM, Plata A, et al. Troisier sign and Virchow node: the anatomy and pathology of pulmonary adenocarcinoma metastasis to a supraclavicular lymph node. Autops Case Rep 2019;9(1). https://doi.org/10.4322/acr.2018.053.

53. Ellison DE, Canalis RF. Sarcoidosis of the head and neck. Clin Dermatol 1986; 4(4):136–42.

54. Badhey AK, Kadakia S, Carrau RL, et al. Sarcoidosis of the Head and Neck. Head Neck Pathol 2015;9(2):260–8.

55. Ungprasert P, Ryu JH, Matteson EL. Clinical Manifestations, Diagnosis, and Treatment of Sarcoidosis. Mayo Clin Proc Innov Qual Outcomes 2019;3(3):358–75.

56. Campbell SM, Montanaro A, Bardana EJ. Head and neck manifestations of autoimmune disease. Am J Otolaryngol Neck Med Surg 1983;4(3):187–216.

57. Doghramji PP. Screening and Laboratory Diagnosis of Autoimmune Diseases Using Antinuclear Antibody Immunofluorescence Assay and Specific Autoantibody Testing. Educational resource.

An Update on Nontumorous Disorders of the Salivary Glands and Their Management for Internists

Kelly E. Daniels, MD, Barry M. Schaitkin, MD*

KEYWORDS

- Sialendoscopy • Salivary glands • Botulinum • Botox • Sialadenitis
- Minimally invasive • Gland-preserving

KEY POINTS

- A diverse set of etiologies can lead to salivary gland disease that is isolated or diffuse and make it a common medical complaint.
- Salivary function is an important contributor to oral health, and lack of intervention for salivary complaints can lead to increased dental caries, bacteremia, and eventually systemic disease.
- Treatment historically involved excision of the gland surgically, an operation that inherently compromised function and carried the risk of complications including nerve injury and sialocele.
- Today's treatment paradigm has shifted to gland-preserving techniques, specifically through the use of sialendoscopy (salivary endoscopy) and injection with botulinum toxin.
- Treatment of many salivary complaints can now be done in the office under local anesthesia or through outpatient operating room procedures that maintain function while minimizing risk of complications and treatment-associated morbidity.

INTRODUCTION, HISTORY, DEFINITIONS, AND BACKGROUND

The major salivary glands include the paired parotid, submandibular, and sublingual glands (**Table 1**). There are also diffusely dispersed minor salivary glands along the buccal mucosal surfaces of the oral cavity. Medical complaints involving these glands range from pathology affecting a single gland to disease that is diffuse and systemic. Etiologies are frequently divided into those that are obstructive, interfering with the normal flow of saliva, and those that are inflammatory, leading to gland dysfunction and destruction. Salivary pathology should be included in the differential when a

University of Pittsburgh Medical Center, 203 Lothrop Street, 5th Floor, Pittsburgh, PA 15213, USA
* Corresponding author.
E-mail address: Schaitkinb@upmc.edu

Med Clin N Am 105 (2021) 839–847
https://doi.org/10.1016/j.mcna.2021.05.006
0025-7125/21/© 2021 Elsevier Inc. All rights reserved.

Table 1	
Quick reference of key terms	
Term	Definition
Sialendectomy	Excision of salivary glands; previously the gold standard
Sialography	An earlier form of salivary duct imaging that involved intravenous contrast and high doses of radiation
Sialendoscopy	A newer form of semirigid scope technology that allows for direct visualization of intraductal tissue and pathology
Sialadenitis	Inflammation of the salivary glands, may be acute vs chronic, often presents as periprandial pain
Sialadenosis	Noninflammatory enlargement or swelling of salivary glands, nontender
Sialolithiasis	Salivary stones, an obstructive process
Sialorrhea	Hypersecretion of saliva
Xerostomia	Hyposecretion of saliva
Drooling	A result of muscle incoordination; quantity and quality of saliva is normal

patient presents with periprandial pain or discomfort that localizes to the head and neck, which are classic obstructive symptoms, or extremes in secretion including too much (sialorrhea) or too little saliva production (xerostomia). Evaluation begins with a thorough history and physical examination and may require additional imaging. Treatment options, depending on the cause, include medical management; gland resection; and more recently, minimally invasive methods, such as endoscopy and botulinum toxin A (Botox) injection.

Historically total gland resection, or sialoadenectomy, was used as definitive treatment of salivary complaints; however, this procedure was associated with complications including nerve damage (for the submandibular gland; the lingual, marginal mandibular, or hypoglossal nerves; and the facial and greater auricular nerves for the parotid gland), salivary fistula, sialocele, and aesthetic issues. Initially introduced in the 1990s, minimally invasive methods, such as sialendoscopy, allow for visualization and intervention while still preserving function.[1,2] Today, as these methods are used more widely, otolaryngologists are able to treat the salivary complaint with a lower risk of these complications, and oftentimes this is done outpatient with sedation or in the office under local anesthesia. This update for internists covers an overview of salivary gland pathologies, with an emphasis on recent treatment advances that has allowed otolaryngologists to relieve symptoms while retaining gland function.

THE ROLE OF SALIVARY DISEASE IN A PERSON'S TOTAL HEALTH

Salivary disease often initially presents with symptoms that are bothersome, but not debilitating. However, it is important to consider the possible downstream outcomes and greater impact on total health for a patient with untreated salivary disease. Chronic oral inflammation and discomfort can lead to dental caries and poor nutrition resulting from decreased or altered saliva.[3]

NATURE OF THE PROBLEM

One of the broadest categories of salivary disease is sialadenitis, and it is helpful to consider it as either obstructive or inflammatory. Obstructive sialadenitis results most frequently from the presence of sialoliths, or stones in the salivary glands, or the presence of a scar, or stenosis of the salivary ductal system. Salivary stones most often occur in the submandibular gland, whereas the parotid gland is more frequently involved in ductal stenosis. These obstructive etiologies frequently present as periprandial discomfort; however, they also can be painless. Salivary stones may be entirely asymptomatic and discovered only incidentally on unrelated imaging. This occurs because the stones grow rather slowly, and as long as they are freely floating in the duct the salivary flow is not obstructed.

Inflammatory causes of sialadenitis often cause bilateral and multiglandular disease, making their presentation unique from obstructive processes. These inflammatory causes can be part of a larger systemic metabolic or autoimmune process, as with Sjögren syndrome, or are isolated to the salivary glands, as with juvenile recurrent parotitis. Inflammation to the glands can also be an iatrogenic side effect of prior radioactive iodine treatment or radiation exposure to the head and neck area. In these processes, there is recurrent inflammation leading to hypofunction of the salivary glands. This hyposecretion leads to xerostomia and salivary stasis, resulting in mucus plugging and duct stenosis, with duct dilation proximal to the stenoses. A variety of causes can lead to inflammatory sialadenitis, listed in **Box 1**. There is also idiopathic chronic sialadenitis, which results in the same pattern of ductal stenosis and dilation; however, this is often limited to a single gland.[4]

Other salivary conditions include sialadenosis. Like inflammatory sialadenitis, sialadenosis is associated with systemic conditions thus leading to bilateral disease. The glandular swelling and hypertrophy characteristic of sialadenosis is associated with disorders affecting the body's metabolism, including anorexia, bulimia, alcoholism,

---

Box 1
Systemic disease processes that are associated with bilateral salivary gland inflammation

Disease or Exposure

Sarcoid

Sjögren syndrome

HIV

Tuberculosis

Gout

Heerfordt syndrome

Bone marrow transplant

Chronic kidney disease on hemodialysis

Malnutrition/vitamin deficiencies

Cystic fibrosis

Diabetes mellitus

Transplant patients: graft-versus-host disease

Chemotherapy

Drug-induced

Viral

IgG4 disease

and cirrhosis.[5] It generally presents with markedly enlarged parotid glands. It is occasionally painful but does not change the quantity or quality of saliva.

OBSERVATION, ASSESSMENT, AND EVALUATION

For patients presenting with a salivary complaint, it is important to obtain a thorough and systemic history. As with any chief complaint, the patient should be asked to characterize the onset and consistency of their presenting symptoms and the exact location or gland involved. The timing of symptoms in relation to mealtime is important to note. Patients with an obstructive cause often present with recurrent periprandial pain, swelling, or discomfort. It is also pertinent to have the patient try to localize their source of discomfort, because isolated versus multiglandular disease is vital to the differential. Patients with an inflammatory cause are more likely to have bilateral disease, with gland swelling or complaints of dry mouth.

Given the range of causes from isolated to pervasive, it is essential to review the patient's complete past medical history with an emphasis on any autoimmune or inflammatory conditions, or any previous radiation exposure. Tobacco use, caffeine use, diabetes, gout, and chronic dehydration can also increase a patient's risk of developing either obstructive or inflammatory sialdenitis.[4] Key elements of the history are highlighted in **Table 2**. The physical examination should include a full otolaryngologic head and neck examination. Following a complete history and physical, conservative management for salivary complaints starts with hydration, sialagogues, warm compresses, and massage. If there are signs of infection, a course of antibiotics may be necessary. For patients failing conservative treatment, further work-up in indicated.

IMAGING

Imaging may be indicated for evaluation. If there is concern for a mass or tumor, an MRI is best for characterizing these lesions. Otherwise, computed tomography is the preferred scan to visualize calcifications, bony erosion, or inflammatory processes including abscesses. Computed tomography with fine cuts with and without contrast is often the imaging of choice for suspected stones. Ultrasound is adequate to visualize masses, lymphadenopathy, stones, obstruction, or dilatation, but may be insufficient to evaluate processes affecting deeper portions of the gland.

GLAND-PRESERVING TREATMENT OPTIONS FOR SALIVARY SYMPTOMS
Sialendoscopy

Sialendoscopy, involving a semirigid salivary lens from 1.1 to 1.6 mm in diameter attached to a camera, allows direct visualization of the salivary ductal collecting system. This procedure is diagnostic and therapeutic in some cases. Sialendoscopy allows the clinician to directly visualize the gland and intervene endoscopically to remove small sialoliths (salivary stones); dilate areas of stenosis; or inject therapeutic medications, such as steroids or Botox. In the appropriate clinical scenario sialendoscopy can be performed in the office under local anesthesia. For patients with more complex disease or whom cannot tolerate the procedure in clinic, sialendoscopy is performed in the operating room under general anesthesia. Outcomes from either setting are comparable.[6]

Sialendoscopy has enabled a new paradigm for the treatment of sialolithiasis. Once requiring gland excision, these stones can now be selectively removed. Small stones are identified and removed using sialendoscopy and endoscopic interventions alone. Larger stones are visualized using sialendoscopy, and then based on their size, shape,

Table 2
Key elements of a patient's history to narrow down a differential diagnosis involving salivary pathology

History	Characteristic	Associated Diagnoses
History of present illness		
	Timing	
	Acute	Infectious
	Chronic	Inflammatory
	Pain	
	Painful	Infection/inflammation, cancer
	Painless	Cancer, sialadenosis
	Worsened by eating?	
	Yes	Sialadenitis
	No	Sialadenosis
	Sidedness	
	Unilateral	Masses, obstructive causes
	Bilateral	Viral parotitis, systemic disease, HIV, malnutrition, metabolic diseases
Review of symptoms		
	Constitutional/fever/chills	Viral (EBV, HIV)
Past medical history		
	Exposure to	
	Radioactive iodine	Xerostomia
	Radiation therapy	Sialadenitis
	Smoking	Warthin tumor
	Unvaccinated (specifically MMR)	Sialadenosis, viral sialadenitis
	Systemic diseases	
	Granulomatous diseases	Sialadenitis
	Sarcoid	Parotid enlargement, sialadenosis
	Sjögren syndrome	Xerostomia, sialadenosis
	Tuberculosis	Unilateral granulomatous disease
	Gout	Sialolithiasis

Abbreviations: EBV, Epstein-Barr virus; MMR, measles, mumps, and, rubella vaccine.

and location can either be surgically excised or fragmented using lithotripsy.[7] Surgical approaches vary with parotid versus submandibular disease based on the relative anatomy, but in both instances sialendoscopy is used to precisely locate the stone thus optimizing surgical approach.[8] Lithotripsy traditionally describes extracorporeal shock waves to fragment a stone, but novel techniques use a hybrid approach with sialendoscopy-directed intraductal lasers or pneumatic devices to fragment the stone and then retrieve pieces using endoscopic tools.[9–11] This treatment paradigm in illustrated in **Fig. 1**.

Stenosis is the second most common obstructive cause. Sialendoscopy has made it possible to differentiate inflammatory stenosis from fibrotic stenosis through direct visualization of the tissue, thus guiding treatment. Inflammatory stenosis is treated with steroids and cortisone irrigations, often guided by sialendoscopy to target

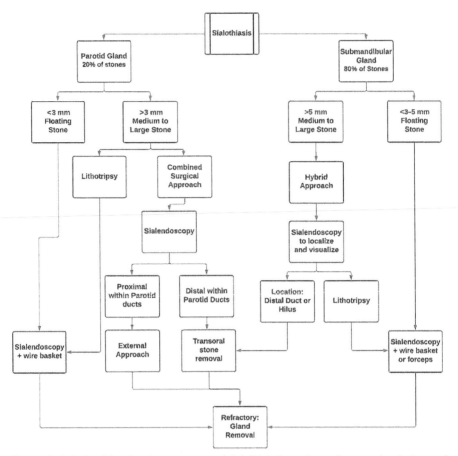

Fig. 1. Clinical algorithm for the treatment of sialolithiasis, as dependent on gland, size, and location.

affected areas. Fibrotic stenosis involves scar tissue in the ductal system, and although it may resolve with cortisone injections it often requires instrumentation to release the stenosis.[1] When stenosis is left untreated, it can lead to irreversible damage of the gland. Prompt treatment allows for the salivary tissue to recover and preserves its function.

Botox

Botox has emerged as an effective treatment of a variety of salivary complaints, and like sialendoscopy, has provided patients with an alternative treatment that is less invasive and more function-sparing than traditional surgical approaches. Botox functions through the drug's irreversible binding to the neural channel protein that is responsible for transporting acetylcholine to the synaptic cleft on the presynaptic cell. In this way, it blocks the release of acetylcholine, thus inhibiting conduction of the neural signal.[12] These channel proteins are eventually replaced, making the effects of Botox transient in nature, lasting an average of 3 months. The temporary effect of Botox lends itself to its pros and cons. The need for serial treatments can make compliance a challenge. However, this also makes it easier to titrate doses to optimize treatments, limits the duration of adverse side effects, and makes Botox a safe way to test efficacy for longer-term or irreversible treatments. Botox has been used in adults and children and has maximum dosage guidelines for both populations. Several of these uses are discussed next.

Sialadenosis describes the hypertrophy of salivary acinar tissue and the resultant typically nontender swelling of salivary glands. If painful, it is thought to be caused by obstruction and stasis occurring. Botox injection with or without additional salivary endoscopy, irrigation, and dilation can control these symptoms. Botox is able to exert an anticholinergic effect blocking the secretomotor stimulation of this glandular tissue. Likewise, Botox injection has been found to improve sialoceles.[13,14] A sialocele is defined as a saliva-containing cavity, which results from trauma to the salivary ductal network disrupting its normal outflow and allowing it to accumulate. This is caused by penetrating trauma or iatrogenically from parotid or submandibular gland surgery. By injecting these pockets and the adjacent salivary tissue with Botox, saliva production is decreased, which allows the aberrant collecting channels to close. Furthermore, Botox can actually shrink the gland by inhibiting the secretory tissues allowing them to atrophy, also yielding positive aesthetic results. Botox lasts longer on autonomic neurons than on muscular tissue and can provide symptoms relief for 5 to 12 months in some instances.[5]

Botox has also proven effective in the treatment of drooling, a condition resulting from a lack of muscle coordination that leads to oral secretions pooling in the mouth. It is important to differentiate drooling from sialorrhea, the condition where the actual quantity and quality of saliva are altered. Drooling is often seen in patients with neurologic impairment, where their swallow is uncoordinated. The impaired clearance of secretions can result in skin breakdown and infection, and impact social interactions and care management. Historically, treatment options included surgical excision of the submandibular glands, or transposition of Wharton duct, both invasive procedures with limited efficacy. A prospective study on Botox injections was conducted in this population. Three months after receiving ultrasound-guided Botox injections to the four major salivary glands, 85% of patients' parents surveyed noticed significant improvement in symptoms, and 88% of them said they would do it again.[15] Most importantly for this patient population, Botox injections were found to be not only efficacious, but also safe and no significant side effects were reported.

After head and neck surgery involving the parapharyngeal space or the parotid gland, patients may develop a painful but usually transient condition called first bite syndrome. This syndrome involves intense pain, originating in the muscles of mastication on the initiation of chewing and radiating to the ear. This sensation lessens in intensity with subsequent bites, making it the worst at the beginning of a meal, and often causing patients to limit their food intake. Although the condition is only temporary, it occurs in up to 18% of patients with parapharyngeal space surgery and proper nutrition is essential in these postoperative patients for wound healing.[16] In a small study, Botox injections have been found to reduce symptoms in 60% of patients, thus providing a low-risk temporizing measure to allow symptoms to be addressed while waiting for the condition to self-resolve.

COMPLICATIONS TO TREATMENT OF SALIVARY COMPLAINTS

Historically, surgical intervention was the standard for medically refractory sialadenitis and carried the risk of salivary fistulas, hypertrophic scarring, infection, hematoma, sialocele, and cutaneous paresthesia. In addition, parotid gland surgery caries the risk of facial paresis, either transiently (25%–55%) or permanently (1%–3%), or Frey syndrome (8%–33%), whereas submandibular gland removal risks injury to the marginal mandibular, hypoglossal, or lingual nerves (1%–8%).[4] With salivary endoscopy, the greatest risk is that of salivary duct perforation, which resolves in 2 weeks. Botox is generally considered low risk when used within the appropriate dosing guidelines, and adverse outcomes are rare and temporary, including transient mild dysphagia.

SUMMARY

It was once believed that a salivary gland that developed a stone was irreversibly damaged. The realization that once the pathology is removed or reversed, these glands can return to normal function has incentivized otolaryngologists to strive to preserve salivary glands whenever possible. The advancement of the sialendoscope in 1995 and novel applications of Botox has drastically changed the treatment paradigm for salivary disease and resulted in improved patient outcomes with vastly decreased morbidity. Today, salivary disease remains common and diverse, but otolaryngologists have a stronger and more effective armamentarium for definitively treating these burdensome symptoms and improving quality life and oral health in patients.

CLINICS CARE POINTS

- Salivary disorders often present as pain or swelling localized to the parotid or submandibular glands, or as chronic dry mouth and oral pain.
- The differential for salivary diseases considers symptoms, laterality, and comorbid conditions or environmental exposures.
- Diagnosis is made by clinical history, physical examination, and imaging or sialendoscopy.
- Salivary complaints can first be addressed conservatively with sialagogues, warm compresses, massage, and antibiotics if there is an infection.
- Patients should be referred to an otolaryngologist if the clinician suspects they are suffering a salivary gland–related complaint that has been refractory to conservative treatment.
- Minimally invasive diagnostic sialendoscopy is performed to determine the cause of the symptoms and determine gland-preserving treatment options. Often sialendoscopy allows for simultaneous therapeutic intervention.
- Resolution of these conditions allows the gland to recover and preserve its function. Prompt treatment, before irreversible tissue damage or scar formation, ensures the best outcome for patients.

DISCLOSURE

The authors have nothing to disclose.

REFERENCES

1. Koch M, Iro H. Salivary duct stenosis: diagnosis and treatment. Acta Otorhinolaryngol Ital 2017;37(2):131–41.
2. Gillespie MB, Walvekar RR, Schaitkin BM, et al. Gland-Preserving Salivary Surgery A Problem-Based Approach. 1st edition. Heidelberg, Germany: Springer; 2018.
3. Meurman JH, Grönroos L. Oral and dental health care of oral cancer patients: hyposalivation, caries and infections. Oral Oncol 2010;46(6):464–7.
4. Vashishta R, Gillespie MB. Salivary endoscopy for idiopathic chronic sialadenitis. Laryngoscope 2013;123(12):3016–20.

5. Karapantzou C, Jakob M, Canis M. Neurotoxin injection in benign submandibular gland hypertrophy: a first choice treatment. Laryngoscope Investig Otolaryngol 2020;5(2):217–20.
6. Coniglio AJ, Deal AM, Bhate O, et al. In-office versus operating room sialendo-scopy: comparison of outcomes, patient time burden, and charge analysis. Otolaryngol Head Neck Surg 2019;160(2):255–60.
7. Matsunobu T, Kurioka T, Miyagawa Y, et al. Minimally invasive surgery of sialoli-thiasis using sialendoscopy. Auris Nasus Larynx 2014;41(6):528–31.
8. Gillespie MB. Combined parotid techniques. Atlas Oral Maxillofac Surg Clin North Am 2018;26(2):133–43.
9. Koch M, Schapher M, Mantsopoulos K, et al. Intraductal pneumatic lithotripsy af-ter extended transoral duct surgery in submandibular sialolithiasis. Otolaryngol Head Neck Surg 2019;160(1):63–9.
10. Capaccio P, Torretta S, Pignataro L, et al. La litotrissia salivare nell'era della scia-loendoscopia. Acta Otorhinolaryngol Ital 2017;37(2):113–21.
11. Guenzel T, Hoch S, Heinze N, et al. Sialendoscopy plus laser lithotripsy in sialo-lithiasis of the submandibular gland in 64 patients: a simple and safe procedure. Auris Nasus Larynx 2019;46(5):797–802.
12. Verheyden J, Blitzer A. Other noncosmetic uses of BOTOX. Disease-a-Month 2002;48(5):357–66.
13. Jeffe JS, Sulman CG. The use of botulinum toxin B in the treatment of a post-traumatic sialocele in a 4-year-old child: a case report. Int J Pediatr Otorhinolar-yngol 2015;79(12):2446–9.
14. Tighe D, Williams M, Howett D. Treatment of iatrogenic sialoceles and fistulas in the parotid gland with ultrasound-guided injection of botulinum toxin A. Br J Oral Maxillofac Surg 2015;53(1):97–8.
15. Alvarenga A, Campos M, Dias M, et al. BOTOX-A injection of salivary glands for drooling. J Pediatr Surg 2017;52(8):1283–6.
16. Ghosh A, Mirza N. First bite syndrome: our experience with intraparotid injections with botulinum toxin type A. Laryngoscope 2016;126(1):104–7.

Manifestations of Human Papillomavirus in the Head and Neck

Cortney Dable, BS, Elizabeth Nicolli, MD*

KEYWORDS

- Human papillomavirus (HPV) • Oropharyngeal cancer (OPC)
- Head and neck cancer (HNC) • Recurrent respiratory papillomatosis (RRP)
- Benign papilloma

KEY POINTS

- Human papillomavirus (HPV) can cause both benign and malignant disease of the head and neck, with the former associated with strains 6 and 11 and the latter with strains 16 and 18.
- Transmissibility of HPV-positive head and neck cancers is related to oral sex and is common among white, middle-aged men.
- Risk factors for developing HPV-positive head and neck squamous cell carcinoma include increased lifetime sexual partners and marijuana usage.
- HPV-positive head and neck cancers are most likely to present with an asymptomatic neck mass and often require extensive workup to establish diagnosis and a multidisciplinary team for management.
- The Gardasil 9 vaccine has been approved by the Food and Drug Administration for the prevention of oropharyngeal head and neck cancers caused by HPV.

INTRODUCTION

Human papillomavirus (HPV) is the most common sexually transmitted infection in the United States.[1] Most of these infections are asymptomatic and resolve spontaneously; however, a small subset remain persistently infected.

HPV is a double-stranded DNA that has more than 200 different variants.[1] Low-risk types such as 6 and 11 cause benign abnormalities such as warts and respiratory tract papillomas. High-risk types 16 and 18 are oncogenic and can lead to cervical, anal, and oropharyngeal cancers.[1] HPV is most commonly transmitted to the head and neck via oral-genital contact. However, reports have suggested that HPV may be

Department of Otolaryngology, University of Miami Miller School of Medicine, 1121 Northwest 14th Street, Sylvester Medical Office Building, 3rd, Floor Suite 325, Miami, FL 33136, USA
* Corresponding author.
E-mail address: exn164@med.miami.edu

Med Clin N Am 105 (2021) 849–858
https://doi.org/10.1016/j.mcna.2021.05.007
0025-7125/21/Published by Elsevier Inc.

transmitted via alternate mechanisms, including open-mouthed kissing, autoinoculation from genital HPV infection, and maternal breastfeeding.[2–4]

Nononcogenic Human Papillomavirus

Low-risk strains of HPV can cause nononcogenic diseases of the head and neck. Recurrent respiratory papillomatosis (RRP) is a condition caused by low-risk HPV strains 6 and 11.[5] In this disease, benign papillomas grow in the respiratory tract, especially the larynx (**Fig. 1**). RRP can be classified as either juvenile-onset, which is transmitted via the mother during childbirth, or adult-onset, which is transmitted through sexual contact. The most common symptom of RRP is hoarseness, but more severe symptoms can exist. Difficulty breathing is one of the more severe symptoms of RRP caused by airway blockage from the lesion and tends to occur more frequently in the juvenile population.[6] The papillomas that typically develop are noncancerous, but generally require multiple surgeries for removal, as they tend to recur.[7] Infection with HPV-11 may have worse outcomes in RRP than HPV-6, as patients with HPV-11 develop more aggressive disease, require more surgeries, and have an increased likelihood of tracheal disease and tracheotomy.[8]

There are also benign papillomas that can exist in the oral cavity and pharynx. These are typically squamous cell papillomas caused by HPV-6 and -11.[9] Most of these lesions occur on the palate, tongue, and lips as a papillary, exophytic nodule with a pedunculated attachment but can present anywhere in the oropharynx.[10–12] These benign papillomas are more common in white men between the third and sixth decade of life.[11,12] They are generally asymptomatic, painless masses that do not necessitate treatment; however, the lesion can be removed via surgery with a scalpel or laser.[13] Once removed, the papillomas usually do not recur.

Oncogenic Human Papillomavirus

Persistent HPV infection with high-risk strains can lead to more aggressive diseases of the head and neck, specifically oropharyngeal cancer (OPC). Historically, head and neck cancers have been associated with tobacco and alcohol use. However, growing literature has shown an increased prevalence of HPV-related head and neck cancer, specifically OPC.[14–16] The most common variant found in head and neck OPC is the high-risk variant HPV-16.[17,18] It is estimated that there are approximately 20,000

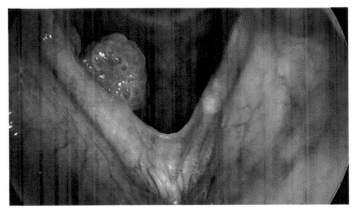

Fig. 1. Recurrent respiratory papillomatosis is caused by HPV strains 6 and 11 and presents as papillomas in the respiratory tract, most commonly the larynx.

new cases of HPV-positive OPC each year, with greater than 80% of cases being men.[19] Increasing awareness of and education about this disease entity is critical to reducing delays in diagnosis and treatment.

Risk Factors for Human Papillomavirus–Related Oropharynx Cancer

Patients with HPV-related OPC do not "look" similar to patients with traditional head and neck cancer. When compared with patients who do not have HPV-positive OPC, they are younger (<60 years), smoke and drink less, and tend to have a higher socio-economic status and higher education level.[20]

The incidence of HPV-positive OPC is highest in white, middle-aged men, with number of lifetime oral sexual partners as the major risk factor.[2,21] It is not entirely clear why there is a higher incidence of HPV-positive OPC in men compared with women. A comparative study found no significant difference in HPV-positive OPC incidence between men and women with 0 to 1 lifetime sexual partners. As lifetime partners increased, there was an increased prevalence of HPV-positive OPC in men compared with women,[22] and this may be secondary to oral sex on a woman being higher risk than oral sex on a man. In addition, men were less likely than women to clear oral HPV infection.[2]

Unlike HPV-negative tumors, tobacco smoking is not a direct cause of HPV-positive OPC.[20] (Although tobacco smoking may lead to worse outcomes in people with HPV-positive OPC, as smoking at diagnosis and during treatment can lead to faster cancer progression, decreased response to treatment, and increased risk of recurrence.).[23] Marijuana use has however been shown to be a risk factor for HPV-positive OPC.[20,24] In 2020 Liu and colleagues described the pathway through which cannabinoid receptors activate cell lines promoting cell growth and migration while inhibiting apoptosis through p38 mitogen-activated protein kinase in HPV-positive OPC[24]; this is especially relevant as more states move to legalize marijuana use.

Workup and Diagnosis

The most common presentation of HPV-positive OPC is an asymptomatic neck mass.[25] Other presenting symptoms may include sore throat or referred otalgia, but these are less common; this is in contrast to HPV-negative OPC, where patients are more likely to present with a sore throat, hoarseness, dysphagia, and odynophagia.[26,27] A lack of these more classic "red flag" cancer symptoms in addition to the lack of traditional risk factors can create a diagnostic challenge for primary care physicians. Furthermore, neck metastases in HPV-positive OPC are often cystic, leading to the misdiagnosis of a branchial cleft cyst in these younger, presumably low-risk patients.[27,28]

The American Academy of Otolaryngology released clinical practice guidelines addressing some of these issues in the evaluation of a neck mass in an adult.[25] A neck mass in an adult patient should be considered malignant until proved otherwise. As in any clinical encounter, the physician should first gather an extensive history. Specifically, one should be asked about symptoms related to head and neck pathology, including, but not limited to, persistent sore throat, otalgia, dysphagia, odynophagia, and hoarseness. A thorough social history should be gathered, including alcohol, marijuana, and tobacco use, as well as lifetime sexual partners and types of sexual activity. If there is nothing in the history to suggest an infectious cause, antibiotics should not be prescribed. Inappropriate treatment with antibiotics is a common cause for delay in diagnosis for these patients.[29,30]

A thorough head and neck examination should be performed. The neck should be inspected and palpated, and the entirety of the oropharyngeal cavity should be examined. When performing the physical examination, special attention should be paid to inspecting and palpating the tonsils and base of tongue due to the high likelihood of HPV-positive cancers being found in these regions. Certain areas of the oropharynx may be difficult to examine, and so referral to otolaryngology should be made, where flexible laryngoscopy can be performed for further inspection of difficult-to-view areas, including the inferior tonsil and base of tongue (**Fig. 2**).

In general, the patient is at increased risk of malignancy if the neck mass persists for longer than 2 weeks and is firm, nonmobile, greater than 1.5 cm, and/or has ulceration.[25] These patients should undergo *contrasted* imaging (either computed tomography [CT] or MRI) (**Fig. 3**). Imaging will help characterize the neck mass as well as evaluate potential primary tumor sites. PET-CT is generally obtained after a confirmed diagnosis of malignancy. It is used primarily for staging but also can be valuable in identifying the primary tumor.

After obtaining an extensive history and physical examination, ultrasound (US)-guided fine-needle aspiration (FNA) should be performed. It has been shown that when combined, US and FNA have a more accurate diagnosis than alone.[31] However, FNA may not be the most useful when determining cytology for HPV-positive OPC. Thus, it is recommended to combine US-guided FNA with concurrent small core biopsy of neck masses and lymph nodes for a more reliable testing of HPV-positive OPC.[32] If a tissue diagnosis cannot be obtained by FNA or small core biopsy, the patient may need to undergo further inspection of the oropharynx with endoscopy under generalized anesthesia.[25] Open biopsies can be performed, but these are only done as a last resort.

In 2017, the World Health Organization recommended direct molecular HPV testing to classify oropharyngeal squamous cell carcinoma types.[33] Furthermore, the College of American Pathologists recommends testing newly diagnosed oropharyngeal

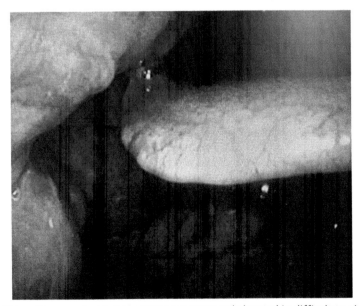

Fig. 2. HPV-positive oropharyngeal cancers are commonly located in difficult-to-view areas, including the inferior tonsil and base of tongue. Flexible laryngoscopy can be performed to better inspect these areas.

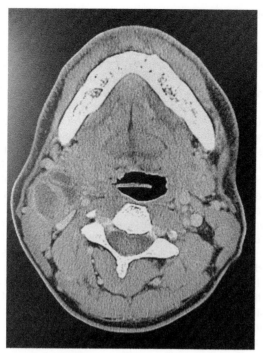

Fig. 3. Neck metastases in HPV-positive oropharyngeal cancers are often cystic; this can be confused with other diseases, including branchial cleft cysts, which can lead to misdiagnosis.

squamous cell carcinoma for high-risk HPV from either the primary site of the tumor or the cervical node metastases.[34] This testing can be done via surrogate marker p16 immunohistochemistry (IHC), as high-risk HPV causes an upregulation of p16. Because IHC only detects p16 and not HPV status, it is usually recommended to confirm a positive p16 IHC with an in situ hybridization (ISH) test.[35] High-risk HPV testing need not be performed on nonsquamous carcinomas or nonoropharyngeal primary tumors of the head and neck.

Treatment and Prognosis

Early diagnosis is important to obtain timely treatment and reduce morbidity and mortality. Once a diagnosis has been established, it is important to have a multidisciplinary team involved. This team should include an otolaryngologist, medical oncologist, and radiation oncologist, as well as a pain management physician, dietician, psychologist, and dentist.[36] Having a multidisciplinary team will lead to better outcomes for the patient, given the complexity of treatment. Treatment involves radiation, chemoradiation, surgery, or some combination of all three. Much of the treatment regimen is dictated by the staging of the cancer, site of disease, patient preferences, hospital volume, and the geographic region.[37]

HPV-positive OPC has better survival rates compared with HPV-negative OPC, with the 3-year survival rates being 82.4% and 57.1%, respectively.[38] Because these patients are younger at diagnosis and have a higher likelihood of cure, there will ultimately be more patients living with the long-term side effects of treatment. Common long-term side effects include depression, anxiety, dysphagia, xerostomia, hypothyroidism, all of which may require primary care intervention.[39]

Screening and Prevention

Currently, there is no recommended screening for HPV-positive OPC.[40] Even though the prevalence of HPV infection is high, the development of OPC among those with HPV infection is low.[41] Therefore, the best current measure to reduce the risk of HPV-positive OPC is prevention by vaccination against HPV.

There are currently 3 vaccines that are licensed by the Food and Drug Administration (FDA) for use in the United States for prevention of HPV-related diseases. These vaccines include Cervarix, which targets HPV-16 and -18; Gardasil, which targets HPV-6, -11, -16, and -18; and Gardasil 9, which targets HPV-6, -11, -16, -18, -31, -33, -45, -53, and -58. All 3 vaccines prevent against the high-risk HPV strains: 16 and 18. Gardasil 9 is currently the only vaccine being distributed in the United States because it offers protection against more strains of HPV than the other vaccines.[42]

Originally, the vaccines for HPV were approved to protect against cervical cancer, because HPV-16 and -18 cause approximately 70% of all cervical cancers.[43] It has since been shown that the vaccine also provides protection from HPV-positive OPC, especially because most of these cancers are caused by the HPV-16 variant.[44] The FDA recently approved Gardasil 9 specifically for prophylaxis of HPV-positive oropharyngeal and other head and neck cancers.[45]

Because of the higher prevalence of HPV-positive OPC in men, it is recommended that men receive the Gardasil 9 vaccine to prevent development of this cancer later on.[46] There may still be some hesitancy, as HPV has been more implicated in women in the past due to the nature of HPV and cervical cancer. However, it is now known that HPV affects the head and neck, so it is important to receive the vaccine as a prophylactic agent.

The guidelines have recently been updated in regard to the logistics of receiving the Gardasil 9 vaccine. According to the Advisory Committee on Immunization Practices (ACIP), the HPV vaccine should be administered in a 2-dose schedule if first given before the age of 15 years and a 3-dose schedule if after the age of 15 years. The one exception for this schedule is patients with human immunodeficiency virus or an immunocompromised state, in which the patient should receive the 3-dose schedule regardless of age.[47]

The recommended age of first receiving the vaccine is around ages 11 to 12 years, but the vaccine can be given as early as 9 years old. The vaccine is recommended to be given to both men and women at an earlier age before any acquired HPV infection. If patients do not start vaccination by age 11 to 12 years, then they should receive catch-up vaccination through 26 years old.[47] Patients aged between 27 and 45 years who have not started or completed HPV vaccination may still be eligible to receive the vaccine.

SUMMARY

Human papillomavirus is the most common sexually transmitted infection in the United States. Persistent infection can lead to various head and neck manifestations, mostly through oral-genital transmission. Nononcogenic strains can cause benign papillomas of the upper aerodigestive tract. High-risk strains can lead to HPV-related oropharyngeal squamous cell carcinoma.

It is most commonly seen in middle-aged men and is related to increased lifetime oral sexual partners and marijuana usage. Unlike HPV-negative OPC, HPV-positive OPC is not directly related to tobacco smoking, alcohol usage, or poor oral hygiene. These patients often present with an asymptomatic neck mass, and thus a high index of suspicion is required to ensure prompt diagnosis. Vaccination against HPV is the best means of prevention.

CLINICS CARE POINTS

- Patients with HPV-related OPC are likely to be middle-aged white men with little to no smoking or drinking history. Number of oral sex partners is the biggest risk factor.
- The most common presentation of HPV-related OPC is an asymptomatic neck mass.
- Vaccination for HPV-positive OPC with Gardasil 9 has recently been recommended by the FDA. Internists can administer these vaccines to patients as early as 9 years old. It is important to educate parents and patients on the importance of receiving this vaccine for cancer prevention.

DISCLOSURE

The authors have nothing to disclose.

REFERENCES

1. Meites E, Gee J, Unger E, et al. Epidemiology and prevention of vaccine-Preventable diseases. Center for Disease Control and Prevention; 2020. Available at: https://www.cdc.gov/vaccines/pubs/pinkbook/hpv.html#:~:text=Studies%20of%20newly%20acquired%20HPV,were%20caused%20by%20HPV%2016. Accessed: March 28, 2021.
2. D'Souza G, Agrawal Y, Halpern J, et al. Oral sexual behaviors associated with prevalent oral human papillomavirus infection. J Infect Dis 2009;199(9):1263–9.
3. Visalli G, Currò M, Facciolà A, et al. Prevalence of human papillomavirus in saliva of women with HPV genital lesions. Infect Agent Cancer 2016;11(1):48.
4. Yoshida K, Furumoto H, Abe A, et al. The possibility of vertical transmission of human papillomavirus through maternal milk. J Obstet Gynaecol 2011;31(6):503–6.
5. Rabah R, Lancaster WD, Thomas R, et al. Human Papillomavirus-11-associated Recurrent Respiratory Papillomatosis is more Aggressive than Human Papillomavirus-6-associated Disease. Pediatr Dev Pathol 2001;4(1):68–72.
6. National Institute on Deafness and Other Communciation Disorders. Recurrent respiratory papillomatosis or laryngeal papillomatosis. Bethesda, Maryland: National Institutes of Health; 2017. Available at: https://www.nidcd.nih.gov/health/recurrent-respiratory-papillomatosis.
7. Armstrong LR, Derkay CS, Reeves WC. Initial results from the national registry for juvenile-onset recurrent respiratory papillomatosis. RRP Task Force. Arch Otolaryngol Head Neck Surg 1999;125(7):743–8.
8. Wiatrak BJ, Wiatrak DW, Broker TR, et al. Recurrent respiratory papillomatosis: a longitudinal study comparing severity associated with human papilloma viral types 6 and 11 and other risk factors in a large pediatric population. Laryngoscope 2004;114(11 Pt 2 Suppl 104):1–23.
9. Major T, Szarka K, Sziklai I, et al. The characteristics of human papillomavirus DNA in head and neck cancers and papillomas. J Clin Pathol 2005;58(1):51–5.
10. Zeuss MS, Miller CS, White DK. In situ hybridization analysis of human papillomavirus DNA in oral mucosal lesions. Oral Surg Oral Med Oral Pathol 1991;71(6):714–20.
11. Abbey LM, Page DG, Sawyer DR. The clinical and histopathologic features of a series of 464 oral squamous cell papillomas. Oral Surg Oral Med Oral Pathol 1980;49(5):419–28.

12. Frigerio M, Martinelli-Kläy CP, Lombardi T. Clinical, histopathological and immu-nohistochemical study of oral squamous papillomas. Acta Odontol Scand 2015;73(7):508–15.
13. Nammour S, Mobadder ME, Namour A, et al. Success Rate of Benign Oral Squa-mous Papilloma Treatments After Different Surgical Protocols (Conventional, Nd:YAG, CO(2) and Diode 980 nm Lasers): A 34-Year Retrospective Study. Pho-tobiomodul Photomed Laser Surg 2021;39(2):123–30.
14. Syrjänen KJ, Pyrhönen S, Syrjänen SM, et al. Immunohistochemical demonstra-tion of human papilloma virus (HPV) antigens in oral squamous cell lesions. Br J Oral Surg 1983;21(2):147–53.
15. Chaturvedi AK, Engels EA, Pfeiffer RM, et al. Human papillomavirus and rising oropharyngeal cancer incidence in the United States. J Clin Oncol 2011; 29(32):4294–301.
16. Mahal BA, Catalano PJ, Haddad RI, et al. Incidence and Demographic Burden of HPV-Associated Oropharyngeal Head and Neck Cancers in the United States. Cancer Epidemiol Biomarkers Prev 2019;28(10):1660–7.
17. Goodman MT, Saraiya M, Thompson TD, et al. Human papillomavirus genotype and oropharynx cancer survival in the United States of America. Eur J Cancer 2015;51(18):2759–67.
18. Castellsagué X, Alemany L, Quer M, et al. HPV Involvement in Head and Neck Cancers: Comprehensive Assessment of Biomarkers in 3680 Patients. J Natl Cancer Inst 2016;108(6):djv403.
19. Centers for Disease Control and Prevention. U.S. Cancer Statistics: Data Visual-izations. 2020. Available at: https://gis.cdc.gov/Cancer/USCS/DataViz.html. Ac-cessed March 26, 2021.
20. Gillison ML, D'Souza G, Westra W, et al. Distinct risk factor profiles for human papillomavirus type 16-positive and human papillomavirus type 16-negative head and neck cancers. J Natl Cancer Inst 2008;100(6):407–20.
21. D'Souza G, Zhang HH, D'Souza WD, et al. Moderate predictive value of demo-graphic and behavioral characteristics for a diagnosis of HPV16-positive and HPV16-negative head and neck cancer. Oral Oncol 2010;46(2):100–4.
22. Chaturvedi AK, Graubard BI, Broutian T, et al. NHANES 2009-2012 Findings: As-sociation of Sexual Behaviors with Higher Prevalence of Oral Oncogenic Human Papillomavirus Infections in U.S. Men. Cancer Res 2015;75(12):2468–77.
23. Gillison ML, Zhang Q, Jordan R, et al. Tobacco smoking and increased risk of death and progression for patients with p16-positive and p16-negative oropha-ryngeal cancer. J Clin Oncol 2012;30(17):2102–11.
24. Liu C, Sadat SH, Ebisumoto K, et al. Cannabinoids Promote Progression of HPV-Positive Head and Neck Squamous Cell Carcinoma via p38 MAPK Activation. Clin Cancer Res 2020;26(11):2693–703.
25. Pynnonen MA, Gillespie MB, Roman B, et al. Clinical Practice Guideline: Evalua-tion of the Neck Mass in Adults. Otolaryngol Head Neck Surg 2017;157(2_suppl): S1–30.
26. Khalid MB, Ting P, Pai A, et al. Initial presentation of human papillomavirus-related head and neck cancer: A retrospective review. Laryngoscope 2019; 129(4):877–82.
27. Truong Lam M, O'Sullivan B, Gullane P, et al. Challenges in establishing the diag-nosis of human papillomavirus-related oropharyngeal carcinoma. Laryngoscope 2016;126(10):2270–5.

28. Goldenberg D, Begum S, Westra WH, et al. Cystic lymph node metastasis in patients with head and neck cancer: An HPV-associated phenomenon. Head Neck 2008;30(7):898–903.

29. Franco J, Elghouche AN, Harris MS, et al. Diagnostic Delays and Errors in Head and Neck Cancer Patients: Opportunities for Improvement. Am J Med Qual 2017; 32(3):330–5.

30. Lee JJ, Dhepnorrarat C, Nyhof-Young J, et al. Investigating Patient and Physician Delays in the Diagnosis of Head and Neck Cancers: a Canadian Perspective. J Cancer Educ 2016;31(1):8–14.

31. Horvath L, Kraft M. Evaluation of ultrasound and fine-needle aspiration in the assessment of head and neck lesions. Eur Arch Otorhinolaryngol 2019;276(10): 2903–11.

32. Allison DB, Miller JA, Coquia SF, et al. Ultrasonography-guided fine-needle aspiration with concurrent small core biopsy of neck masses and lymph nodes yields adequate material for HPV testing in head and neck squamous cell carcinomas. J Am Soc Cytopathol 2016;5(1):22–30.

33. El-Naggar AK, Chan JK, Grandis JR, et al. WHO classification of head and neck tumours. Lyon, France: International Agency for Research on Cancer (IARC); 2017.

34. Lewis JS Jr, Beadle B, Bishop JA, et al. Human Papillomavirus Testing in Head and Neck Carcinomas: Guideline From the College of American Pathologists. Arch Pathol Lab Med 2018;142(5):559–97.

35. Craig SG, Anderson LA, Schache AG, et al. Recommendations for determining HPV status in patients with oropharyngeal cancers under TNM8 guidelines: a two-tier approach. Br J Cancer 2019;120(8):827–33.

36. Kelly SL, Jackson JE, Hickey BE, et al. Multidisciplinary clinic care improves adherence to best practice in head and neck cancer. Am J Otol 2013;34(1): 57–60.

37. Zhan KY, Puram SV, Li MM, et al. National treatment trends in human papillomavirus-positive oropharyngeal squamous cell carcinoma. Cancer 2020; 126(6):1295–305.

38. Ang KK, Harris J, Wheeler R, et al. Human papillomavirus and survival of patients with oropharyngeal cancer. N Engl J Med 2010;363(1):24–35.

39. Funk GF, Karnell LH, Christensen AJ. Long-term health-related quality of life in survivors of head and neck cancer. Arch Otolaryngol Head Neck Surg 2012; 138(2):123–33.

40. U.S. Preventive Services Task Force. Oral cancer: screening 2013. Available at: https://www.uspreventiveservicestaskforce.org/uspstf/recommendation/oral-cancer-screening. Accessed: March 26, 2021.

41. D'Souza G, McNeel TS, Fakhry C. Understanding personal risk of oropharyngeal cancer: risk-groups for oncogenic oral HPV infection and oropharyngeal cancer. Ann Oncol 2017;28(12):3065–9.

42. Saraiya M, Unger ER, Thompson TD, et al. US Assessment of HPV Types in Cancers: Implications for Current and 9-Valent HPV Vaccines. JNCI. J Natl Cancer Inst 2015;107(6).

43. de Sanjose S, Quint WG, Alemany L, et al. Human papillomavirus genotype attribution in invasive cervical cancer: a retrospective cross-sectional worldwide study. Lancet Oncol 2010;11(11):1048–56.

44. Chaturvedi AK, Graubard BI, Broutian T, et al. Effect of Prophylactic Human Papillomavirus (HPV) Vaccination on Oral HPV Infections Among Young Adults in the United States. J Clin Oncol 2018;36(3):262–7.

45. US Food and Drug Administration. Supplement accelerated approval. 2020. Available at: https://www.fda.gov/media/138949/download. Accessed: March 21, 2021.

46. Graham DM, Isaranuwatchai W, Habbous S, et al. A cost-effectiveness analysis of human papillomavirus vaccination of boys for the prevention of oropharyngeal cancer. Cancer 2015;121(11):1785–92.

47. Oshman LD, Davis AM. Human Papillomavirus Vaccination for Adults: Updated Recommendations of the Advisory Committee on Immunization Practices (ACIP). J Am Med Assoc 2020;323(5):468–9.

Acute and Chronic Sinusitis

Benjamin S. Bleier, MD[a],*, Marianella Paz-Lansberg, MD[b]

KEYWORDS

- Rhinosinusitis • Acute • Chronic • Polyps • Intranasal corticosteroids • Endoscopy
- Surgery

KEY POINTS

- Rhinosinusitis refers to a broadly diverse range of inflammatory conditions affecting the nasal cavity and sinuses and can be classified as either acute or chronic.
- Acute rhinosinusitis in adults is defined as sinonasal inflammation lasting less than 12 weeks and is usually a self-limited condition with a viral cause. Symptoms persisting beyond 7 to 10 days, or still worsening after 5 to 7 days, should likewise raise concern for acute bacterial rhinosinusitis requiring antibiotics.
- Chronic rhinosinusitis (CRS) refers to symptoms persisting longer than 12 weeks and can be broadly divided into 2 phenotypes based on nasal endoscopy and computed tomography findings: CRS without nasal polyps and CRS with nasal polyps. Recent research has primarily focused on refining the understanding of the various CRS biological subtypes (known as endotypes) based on specific pathophysiologic mechanisms and the inflammatory biomarkers of individuals.

INTRODUCTION

The term rhinosinusitis encompasses multiple conditions caused by inflammation of the nasal cavity and sinuses (**Table 1**). The incidence is difficult to estimate given that the clinical manifestations of the disease overlap with some other conditions also affecting the upper respiratory tract. Rhinosinusitis is thought to affect around 31 million people in the United States annually and it is known to significantly affect individual quality of life (QOL) on par with other chronic diseases such as diabetes and congestive heart failure[1] (**Fig. 1**).

ACUTE RHINOSINUSITIS
Definitions and Background of Acute Rhinosinusitis

Acute rhinosinusitis (ARS) in adults is defined by ICAR-RS 2021 as sinonasal inflammation lasting less than 12 weeks and resulting in symptoms such as nasal blockage

[a] Department of Otolaryngology–Head & Neck Surgery, Massachusetts Eye and Ear Infirmary, Harvard Medical School, Boston, MA, USA; [b] Clinical Fellow of Rhinology & Skull Base Surgery, Department of Otolaryngology–Head & Neck Surgery, Massachusetts Eye and Ear Infirmary, Harvard Medical School, 243 Charles Street, Boston, MA 02114, USA
* Corresponding author.
E-mail address: Benjamin_Bleier@MEEI.HARVARD.EDU

Med Clin N Am 105 (2021) 859–870
https://doi.org/10.1016/j.mcna.2021.05.008
0025-7125/21/© 2021 Elsevier Inc. All rights reserved.

medical.theclinics.com

Table 1
Diagnosis summary

Diagnosis	Symptoms	CT Findings	Endoscopy Findings	Symptom Duration
ARS	Nasal blockage/ congestion Or Rhinorrhea/PND And Facial pain/pressure OR Decreased sense of smell	Not necessary	Not necessary	<12 wk
ABRS	Nasal blockage/ congestion OR Rhinorrhea/PND And Facial pain/pressure Or Decreased sense of smell	Not necessary	Not necessary	Persistent after 7–10 d Or Acutely worsening after 5–7 d
RARS	Nasal blockage/ congestion Or Rhinorrhea/PND And Facial pain/pressure Or Decreased sense of smell	Not necessary	Not necessary	>4/y with symptom-free intervals
CRS	>2 of the following: • Nasal blockage/ congestion • Rhinorrhea/PND • Decreased sense of smell • Facial pain/pressure	Evidence of inflammation	Evidence of inflammation And/or Drainage from sinus or OMC (−) Polyps: CRSsNP (+) Polyps: CRSwNP	>12 wk
AECRS	>2 of the following: • Nasal blockage/ congestion • Rhinorrhea/PND • Decreased sense of smell • Facial pain/pressure	Evidence of inflammation	Evidence of inflammation And/or Purulence from sinus or OMC	Acute worsening of symptoms with a return to baseline after treatment

Abbreviations: ABRS, acute bacterial rhinosinusitis; AECRS, acute exacerbation of chronic rhinosinusitis; ARS, acute rhinosinusitis; CRS, chronic rhinosinusitis; CRSsNP, chronic rhinosinusitis without nasal polyposis; CRSwNP: chronic rhinosinusitis with nasal polyposis; CT, computed tomography; OMC, ostiomeatal complex; PND, postnasal drip; RARS, recurrent bacterial rhinosinusitis.

or congestion, anterior nasal discharge, postnasal drip, and facial pain or pressure with or without a decreased sense of smell. ARS is a common entity and accounts for up to 10% of ambulatory care and otolaryngology visits.[2] According to a clinical practice guideline published by the American Academy of Otolaryngology–Head and Neck Surgery in 2015, patients with recurrent episodes of ARS may spend

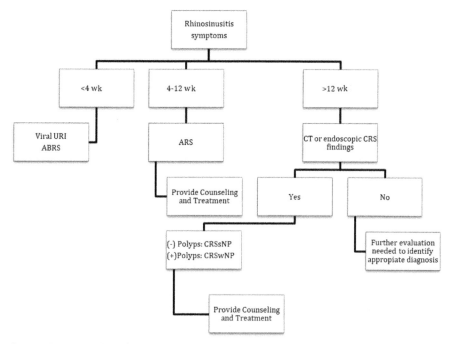

Fig. 1. Diagnostic algorithm. ABRS, acute bacterial rhinosinusitis; ARS, acute rhinosinusitis; CT, computed tomography; CRS, chronic rhinosinusitis; CRSsNP, chronic rhinosinusitis without nasal polyposis; CRSwNP, chronic rhinosinusitis with nasal polyposis; URI, upper respiratory infection.

more than US$1000 yearly in direct treatment costs, in addition to missed workdays and lost productivity.[3]

Most cases of ARS have a viral cause, with a list of potential causes that includes rhinovirus, coronavirus, influenza, parainfluenza, and respiratory syncytial virus.[4] Viral cases are for the most part self-limiting. Situations where symptoms persist after 7 to 10 days, or still worsen acutely 5 to 7 days after initial presentation, should raise concern for acute bacterial rhinosinusitis (ABRS).[3,5] Although the true incidence of acute bacterial ABRS is unknown, it is estimated that less than 2% of ARS cases are bacterial.[2]

The physiopathology of ARS is complex, but the existing literature strongly supports a premise wherein respiratory viruses and bacteria create an inflammatory environment within the nasal and paranasal mucosa, thereby precipitating increased mucus production and a swelling of the nasal and sinus epithelium culminating in the obstruction of the sinus ostia and symptoms such as rhinorrhea, postnasal drip, and facial pressure and discomfort.[4]

The most common bacterial organisms likely to produce ABRS include *Streptococcus pneumoniae*, *Haemophilus influenzae*, and *Moraxella catarrhalis*.[4,6] *Staphylococcus aureus*, although a less common cause, has potentially greater morbidity because it is far more frequently associated with ABRS complications.[4] Within clinical best practice, as currently understood, sinonasal cultures are usually unnecessary at the diagnostic stage and should be reserved for cases where medical treatment seems to be failing.

Prompt recognition and differentiation of these entities is vital in order to provide patients with the best possible course of care, including proper counseling and management.

Diagnosis of uncomplicated ARS is usually a clinical matter, and careful attention to a patient's symptoms and symptomatic timeline should in most cases suffice for accurate diagnosis. Diagnostic imaging testing such as computed tomography (CT) scans or MRI are not usually necessary unless complications such as meningitis, orbital cellulitis, or brain or orbital abscess are present or suspected.[3]

Another important entity to recognize is recurrent acute rhinosinusitis (RARS), which refers to patients that present with 4 or more episodes of ARS per year with symptom-free intervals between each episode. Each episode must meet criteria for ARS and should be treated as such.[2]

Discussion of Treatment Options

Various treatment options for ARS have been extensively discussed in the literature (**Table 2**). Treatments based on current evidence include:

1. Intranasal corticosteroids (INCS) have been shown to ameliorate symptoms, ostensibly by reducing sinonasal inflammation. INCS can be an effective monotherapy in mild to moderate cases or else can be added to an antibiotic course in bacterial cases which, as discussed earlier, are also the most likely to be severe.[2,7] In contrast, systemic corticosteroids have only shown minimal short-term benefits compared with placebo and are not recommended as a potential monotherapy.[2,3]

2. Antibiotic treatment can also be considered for patients with persistent or worsening symptoms a week or longer into treatment. There is some evidence that antibiotics may shorten symptom duration, although their comparative efficacy vis à vis placebo remains small. Such therapy also has well-known side effects, including gastrointestinal issues and weakening of bacterial resistance in the long run.[2,8–10] If antibiotics are ultimately found to be warranted, the most appropriate candidate will be a course of amoxicillin (with or without clavulanate) for a period of 5 to 10 days. In patients with a penicillin allergy, either doxycycline or fluoroquinolones are acceptable alternatives.[3] If a patient being given antibiotics subsequently worsens, or fails to improve within a week, careful reevaluation may be needed to rule out other disorders, ABRS complications, or possible antibiotic-resistant pathogens.

3. Decongestants have been used for many years for treatment of ARS and common colds to relieve uncomfortable nasal congestion and increase patency within blocked sinus ostia. Importantly, topical decongestants may lead to rhinitis medicamentosa with worsening nasal congestion when used for more than 5 consecutive days. Oral decongestants likewise have multiple systemic side effects, including hypertension and tachycardia. As a result, decongestants are generally not recommended as a monotherapy and, if included in a treatment, should always be limited to a shorter period of time.[2,3]

4. Nasal saline irrigations or sprays represent an optional treatment that can help with symptomatic relief of ARS.[2,3] With regard to the choice of hypertonic saline versus normal saline, recent studies have found no significant difference.[2,3]

5. Therapies to avoid:
   a. Antihistamine use in treating ARS is discouraged because it increases dryness within the nasal mucosa, which can ultimately worsen nasal congestion. Although this therapy can in rare cases play a productive role for patients whose

Table 2
Treatment summary

Diagnosis	Management	Recommended	Optional	Not Recommended
ARS	Medical therapy	INCS	• Antibiotics: when ABRS is suspected • Saline sprays/irrigations • Decongestants: only short courses <5 d	• Systemic CS • Antihistamines • Guaifenesin or glyceryl guaiacolate
CRSsNP	Medical therapy	Saline sprays/irrigations Oral antibiotics	INCS Oral CS (only short courses)	• Topical antibiotics • Topical antifungals
	AMT		• Oral antibiotics • Systemic CS	
	Postsurgical management	• Saline spray/irrigations • Sinus cavity debridement • INCS	• CS-eluting implants	
CRSwNP	Medical therapy	Saline spray/irrigations INCS: • Sprays • Irrigations Oral CS (only short courses)	• CS-eluting implants • CS exhalation delivery devices • Antileukotrienes	• Topical antibiotics • Topical antifungals • Nonmacrolide antibiotics <3 wk
	AMT	Biologics (in setting of medical/surgical failure)	Oral antibiotics	—
	Postsurgical management	• Saline spray/irrigations • Sinus cavity debridement • INCS	• Oral antibiotics • Systemic CS • CS-eluting implants	—

Abbreviations: AMT, appropriate medical therapy; CS, corticosteroids; INCS, intranasal corticosteroids.

symptoms support a strong allergic background, such cases remain infrequent and clinicians should generally err on the side of caution.[3]

b. Guaifenesin or glyceryl guaiacolate: is commonly prescribed by medical providers attempting to thin mucosal secretions and lessen patient discomfort. However, this therapy is not recommended for ARS management because its efficacy has not been established.[3]

CHRONIC RHINOSINUSITIS
Definitions and Background of Chronic Rhinosinusitis

Chronic rhinosinusitis (CRS) is a chronic inflammatory disease of the nasal mucosa and paranasal sinuses that severely affects the QOL of those afflicted. It is characterized by the presence of 2 or more of the following symptoms: nasal blockage or congestion, nasal discharge or postnasal drip, hyposmia, or facial pain/pressure. Objective validation of the disease can be obtained by nasal endoscopy or by CT scan showing sinonasal inflammation or evidence of purulent drainage from sinuses or the osteomeatal complex (over a period surpassing 12 weeks in duration).[2,11] CRS is a common condition worldwide, and multiple studies have estimated a prevalence within the US population ranging from 2.1% to 13.8%.[2]

CRS produces significant adverse effects on the QOL and social functioning of individuals with the condition. Notably, QOL surveys have shown that people with CRS scored lower than patients with other chronic conditions such as chronic pain, congestive heart failure, and chronic obstructive pulmonary disease.[2,3] In addition, the annual direct cost to patients for CRS-related medical care and management adds up to more than US$2000 on average, not including the indirect costs of an average 18 missed workdays yearly and decreased average productivity.[3]

In general, medical therapy usually represents the first step in managing CRS, and only when a course of appropriate medical therapy (AMT) fails should surgical treatment in the form of endoscopic sinus surgery (ESS) be seriously considered.[2] Multiple treatment options currently exist and are designed to target the inflammatory chain within the nasal and paranasal mucosa.

Nasal endoscopy and CT scan remain crucial tools for diagnosing CRS. Despite the high prevalence of allergies in patients with rhinosinusitis, allergy testing is not indicated unless the patient reports strong symptoms of allergic rhinitis, such as sneezing, itchy or watery eyes, or rhinorrhea are present. Immune function testing should be reserved for situations where maximal medical management has already failed or where recurrent infections, such as otitis media, bronchiectasis, or pneumonia, are also present.[2,3]

Within the literature, CRS has been broadly divided into 2 main phenotypes based on nasal endoscopy and CT findings: CRS without nasal polyps (CRSsNP) and CRS with nasal polyps (CRSwNP).[2,12] The pathogenesis underlying this condition is likewise known to be more complex than when treating patients based on the phenotypes alone.

Practitioners continue to encounter difficulties in managing patients affected by CRS, especially those with nasal polyposis, because individual response to the same medical or surgical therapies can produce idiosyncratic results. As a result, CRS continues to receive substantial attention from researchers in hopes of better understanding such outcomes. Much of this work to date has focused on better defining the various biological subtypes of CRS, known as endotypes. This classification is based on specific physiologic inflammatory mechanisms and inflammatory biomarkers, characteristics that can vary greatly from individual to individual. Although there is as yet no full consensus as to the specific biomarkers present for each endotype, considerable research supports differentiation rather than the presence of T-helper (Th) 1, Th2, and Th17 inflammatory responses (commonly known as type 1, 2, and 3 immune reactions, respectively.)[2,11,13]

Multiple studies have shown that many patients with CRSwNP show an increased Th2-mediated inflammatory cycle that is characterized by increased eosinophil levels and increased levels of immunoglobulin E, interleukin (IL)-4, IL-5, and IL-13.[13,14] The presence of type 2 versus non–type 2 endotypes presently seems to be the most clinically meaningful such differentiator, because patients with this endotype usually face other inflammatory conditions related to Th2 immune reactions, such as asthma. This observation was notably what initially motivated the use of biologics targeting Th2 inflammation in patients with CRSwNP, and to date this has met with recognizable success.[2,13]

The role of aspirin-exacerbated respiratory disease, also known as Samter's Triad, among patients with CRSwNP also warrants consideration. Patients with this medical condition usually present with asthma, CRSwNP, and sensitivity to aspirin and other nonsteroidal antiinflammatory drugs, known as cyclooxygenase-1 inhibitors. Treatment with aspirin desensitization should be considered after ESS because this approach has been shown to significantly improve safety during desensitization and lessen the risk of aspirin-induced decreased lower airway reactivity.[15]

Another important condition worth flagging is acute exacerbation of chronic rhinosinusitis (AECRS), which refers to the sudden worsening of CRS symptoms with a return to baseline symptoms, often after treatment.[2]

Discussion of Treatment Options

Treatment of CRS is also complex, and considerable challenges remain because, to date, a clear consensus on therapeutic best practices has yet to materialize (see **Table 2**).

Treatment of CRSsNP based on current evidence:

1. INCS sprays are widely recommended and have been shown to improve symptoms and nasal endoscopy score. INCS irrigations may also provide additional benefits to patients after ESS, improving QOL scores, symptom scores, and endoscopic appearance in postoperative patients.[2] INCS use should generally be maintained for a period of at least 8 to 12 weeks before reevaluating treatment success.[3]
2. Nasal saline irrigations or sprays are widely available to patients and are recommended both as monotherapy and as an adjuvant to INCS. Irrigations seem to be significantly more efficient than sprays for clearing secretions. The use of isotonic and hypertonic nasal solutions is largely as a wash, because both have produced similarly results in improving QOL scores and endoscopic sinonasal appearance.[2,3]
3. Antibiotics, specifically a prolonged course of macrolides, seems to improve outcomes on imaging findings, mucus cytokines, and patient-reported symptom score, although consensus regarding treatment dosage and duration remains elusive.[2,3] Topical antibiotics are not recommended.[2,3,16]
4. Topical antifungals are neither beneficial nor recommended.[2,3,17,18]

Treatment of CRSwNP based on current evidence:

1. Oral corticosteroids have long been used to modulate the inflammatory response within the nose and the sinus mucosa, thereby decreasing edema and reducing the size of existing nasal polyps. However, although such treatments can produce

a strong initial mirage response, such results tend not to last once therapy is discontinued.[11] Although they can still be used in conjunction with INCS, it is worth remembering that systemic corticosteroids are nonspecific when targeting inflammation and have well-known adverse effects on the hypothalamic-pituitary-adrenal axis, thus warranting additional caution.[2]

2. INCS are a mainstay for managing patients with CRSwNP, and their use is supported by many studies. INCS have been shown to improve patients' symptoms, improve endoscopy score, decrease polyp size, and forestall polyp recurrence, as well as improve sense of smell and QOL scores. Over the years, multiple routes of steroid administration delivery methods (nasal sprays, irrigations, exhalation delivery system) have been explored for the treatment of nasal polyposis. INCS sprays are widely available and recommended for use as a first step in managing CRSwNP. Multiples studies have shown that topical therapies are effective, and remain relatively safe, showing minimal systemic absorption and minimal effect on cortisol levels. Other forms of INCS administration, such as irrigations, are recommended only in cases where earlier spray therapy has proved insufficient in controlling sinonasal symptoms. In such cases, twice-daily dosing can also represent an intermediate treatment strategy (before irrigation). Some studies have shown that the administering of topical steroids via exhalation delivery systems (EDSs), such as Xhance, can significantly reduce polyp size, improving sinonasal symptoms and QOL scores compared with placebo. EDSs can make for more effective drug delivery within the nasal cavity and sinuses compared with INCS sprays, rendering it a relatively safe option that improves bioavailability.[2,3,19,20]

3. Corticosteroid-eluting implants are widely considered to be the newer alternative for steroid delivery therapy. Implants are placed in patients who have already undergone primary or revision ESS, and these have shown promising results, particularly in decreasing ethmoid sinus obstruction and polyp burden, reducing nasal obstruction scores, and preventing the need for revision ESS. To date, multiple studies have shown no major side effects and there is no evidence of clinically significant increases in intraocular pressure or cataract risk.[2,21,22]

4. Biologics: dupilumab and mepolizumab are biologic therapies that target the Th2 inflammatory response, which plays a key role in the development of nasal polyposis and asthma. Dupilumab is a monoclonal antibody to a subunit of the IL-4 receptor (which inhibits signaling of IL-4 and IL-13). IL-4 is known to have an important immune-response effect on fibroblasts and polyp formation in CRS. Dupilumab has been shown to decrease polyp size and nasal congestion and improve sinus imaging scores, sense of smell, and asthma control. This particular therapy is usually reserved for patients who have already failed prior medical and surgical management or else present with concomitant uncontrolled asthma.[2,13] Mepolizumab is a monoclonal antibody against IL-5 that is known to induce eosinophil proliferation, differentiation, and migration. Anti–IL-5 treatments have shown significant decreases in nasal polyp size, as well as symptom and CT sinus scores in medical studies. Given the comparative expensiveness of mepolizumab and dupilumab, both therapies should be reserved only for select patients whose CRSwNP condition proves resistant to prior medical and surgical therapies.[23]

5. Antibiotics, specifically a prolonged course of macrolide antibiotics lasting longer than 3 weeks, can improve symptom and endoscopic scores in patients with CRSwNP. Some studies have shown decreased polyp size both clinically and on imaging, as well a decrease in IL-8 levels.[24] Macrolides seem to be beneficial, but the appropriate dosage and treatment duration remain unclear. Short-term use of nonmacrolide antibiotic therapy is not recommended for management of

CRSwNP unless there is evidence of an acute exacerbation. Topical antibiotics are likewise not recommended, because randomized control trials have not shown them to be more effective in significant patient improvement than a placebo.[2,11]

6. Antileukotriene use, according to the literature, produces positive effects on patient symptoms similar to INCS and can be considered for patients with CRSwNP instead of, or in addition to, INCS.[2] (This option may warrant particular consideration for juvenile patients because it is available as a chewable tablet.)

7. Topical antifungals, much as is the case for CRSsNP, are not recommended for treatment of CRSwNP. Multiple randomized controlled trials have failed to prove significant improvement of CRS symptoms with topical antifungal therapy compared with placebo.[2,3,17,18]

Surgical Management of Chronic Rhinosinusitis

Surgical management of CRS is usually reserved for patients who have failed to improve after AMT.[2,11] The main goal of ESS in patients with CRS is to create an adequate sinus cavity to allow sinus ventilation and drainage, facilitate mucociliary clearance, and aid in the delivery of postoperative therapies such as saline rinses and INCS.

ESS outcomes in patients with CRS are an area that has been comprehensively assessed within the literature. Multiples studies have clearly shown positive postoperative results with a statistically significant decrease in such CRS symptoms as facial pressure, nasal congestion, nasal obstruction, rhinorrhea, and hyposmia, as well as marked improvements in objective testing scores such as the Sinonasal Outcomes Test-22 (SNOT-22) and QOL questionnaires.[2]

International consensus statement on allergy and rhinology: rhinosinusitis 2021 (ICAR-RS 2021) recommends ESS primarily for patients with CRSsNP and CRSwNP for whom symptoms have failed to improve following 3 to 4 weeks of treatment with INCS and saline irrigations. Oral corticosteroids and/or antibiotic therapies are also likely to be attempted before proceeding with surgery.[2] Likewise, the respective pros and cons of surgery should be carefully discussed with patients on a case-by-case basis, and their personal preferences as well as cost considerations and comorbidity risk should be taken into account.[25]

CRS is a chronic condition and, if a decision is made to proceed with surgery following the failure of medical management, it will be of vital importance to carefully manage patient expectations. This management should include communicating to the patient that surgery does not represent a 1-stop curative solution but is a component part of the ongoing treatment, and one with a nonnegligible ($\approx$16%) chance of requiring additional revision surgeries.[26]

The crucial importance of educating patients about their conditions and likely post-surgical challenges cannot be overstated, because this is key not only to patient satisfaction but also to improving compliance with postoperative medical management, such as saline irrigations and INCS, that facilitates the healing process and enhances CRS symptom reduction in the future.[27,28]

SUMMARY

Rhinosinusitis refers to inflammation of the nasal mucosa and paranasal sinuses. In order to make the appropriate diagnosis, it is important to perform a complete and detailed inquiry not only of the patient's specific symptoms but also of the duration and the larger timeline of the condition. Learning to differentiate with a high degree of certainty between superficially similar sinus conditions such as ARS, ABRS,

RARS, CRSsNP and CRSwNP, and AECRS remains of vital importance. Confident diagnosis, proper counseling, and meticulous medical management skills can together achieve better symptom reduction and improved QOL for patients with these conditions.

CLINICS CARE POINTS

- INCS can be effectively used as a monotherapy for patients with mild to moderate ARS or it can be used in conjunction with antibiotic therapy, the latter usually for more severe cases with persistent or worsening symptoms for longer than 7 days. The antibiotic of first resort should be amoxicillin, with or without clavulanate, although doxycycline or fluoroquinolones can be acceptable alternatives for patients allergic to penicillin. Nasal saline irrigations or sprays can be considered optional but can be added to treatment for symptomatic relief.

- In patients with CRSsNP, INCS can be used to improve most patients' symptoms, and saline irrigations are also recommended both as monotherapy and as an adjuvant to INCS. Although macrolide antibiotics seem to improve patients' outcomes, there is as yet no consensus regarding treatment dosage and duration.

- The use of INCS for patients with CRSwNP is supported by multiple studies, and topical therapies are effective and remain fairly safe. Macrolide antibiotics, when used for longer than 3 weeks, seem to be beneficial even though the appropriate dosage and treatment durations remain unclear. Biologics such as dupilumab and mepolizumab are monoclonal antibodies targeting IL-4 and IL-5 respectively. Both have been shown to decrease polyp size and improve nasal congestion, sinus imaging scores, sense of smell, and asthmatic control. As previously mentioned, these should generally be reserved only for patients who have already failed prior medical and surgical management attempts.

- Surgical management of CRS should likewise be reserved primarily for patients who have exhausted maximal medical therapy and failed to improve. In such cases, careful communication with the patient, both before and after surgical intervention, is key for managing expectations and securing the appropriate delivery of important postoperative therapies such as saline rinses and INCS.

DISCLOSURE

The authors have nothing to disclose.

REFERENCES

1. Benninger MS, Ferguson BJ, Hadley JA, et al. Adult chronic rhinosinusitis: definitions, diagnosis, epidemiology, and pathophysiology. Otolaryngol Head Neck Surg 2003;129(3 Suppl):S1–32.
2. Orlandi RR, Kingdom TT, Smith TL, et al. International Consensus Statement on Allergy and Rhinology: Rhinosinusitis 2021. Int Forum Allergy Rhinol 2021;11(3):213-739.
3. Rosenfeld RM, Piccirillo JF, Chandrasekhar SS, et al. Clinical practice guideline (update): adult sinusitis. Otolaryngol Head Neck Surg 2015;152(2 Suppl):S1–39.
4. Meltzer EO, Hamilos DL, Hadley JA, et al, American Academy of Allergy, Asthma and Immunology (AAAAI), American Academy of Otolaryngic Allergy (AAOA), American Academy of Otolaryngology–Head and Neck Surgery (AAO-HNS), American College of Allergy, Asthma and Immunology (ACAAI), American Rhinologic Society (ARS). Rhinosinusitis: establishing definitions for clinical research and patient care. J Allergy Clin Immunol 2004;114(6 Suppl):155–212.

5. Benninger MS, Sedory Holzer SE, Lau J. Diagnosis and treatment of uncompli- cated acute bacterial rhinosinusitis: summary of the Agency for Health Care Pol- icy and Research evidence-based report. Otolaryngol Head Neck Surg 2000; 122(1):1–7.

6. Benninger M, Brook I, Farrell DJ. Disease severity in acute bacterial rhinosinusitis is greater in patients infected with Streptococcus pneumoniae than in those in- fected with Haemophilus influenzae. Otolaryngol Head Neck Surg 2006;135(4): 523–8.

7. Meltzer EO, Teper A, Danzig M. Intranasal corticosteroids in the treatment of acute rhinosinusitis. Curr Allergy Asthma Rep 2008;8(2):133–8.

8. Sng WJ, Wang DY. Efficacy and side effects of antibiotics in the treatment of acute rhinosinusitis: a systematic review. Rhinology 2015;53(1):3–9.

9. Lemiengre MB, van Driel ML, Merenstein D, et al. Antibiotics for acute rhinosinu- sitis in adults. Cochrane Database Syst Rev 2018;9(9):CD006089.

10. Rosenfeld RM, Singer M, Jones S. Systematic review of antimicrobial therapy in patients with acute rhinosinusitis. Otolaryngol Head Neck Surg 2007;137(3 Suppl):S32–45.

11. Fokkens WJ, Lund VJ, Hopkins C, et al. European position paper on rhinosinusitis and nasal Polyps 2020. Rhinology 2020;58(Suppl S29):1–464.

12. Tan BK, Schleimer RP, Kern RC. Perspectives on the etiology of chronic rhinosi- nusitis. Curr Opin Otolaryngol Head Neck Surg 2010;18(1):21–6.

13. Smith KA, Pulsipher A, Gabrielsen DA, et al. Biologics in chronic rhinosinusitis: an update and thoughts for future directions. Am J Rhinol Allergy 2018;32(5): 412–23.

14. Bachert C, Gevaert P, Holtappels G, et al. Total and specific IgE in nasal polyps is related to local eosinophilic inflammation. J Allergy Clin Immunol 2001;107(4): 607–14.

15. Huang GX, Palumbo ML, Singer JI, et al. Sinus surgery improves lower respira- tory tract reactivity during aspirin desensitization for AERD. J Allergy Clin Immu- nol Pract 2019;7(5):1647–9.

16. Soler ZM, Oyer SL, Kern RC, et al. Antimicrobials and chronic rhinosinusitis with or without polyposis in adults: an evidenced-based review with recommenda- tions. Int Forum Allergy Rhinol 2013;3(1):31–47.

17. Ebbens FA, Georgalas C, Luiten S, et al. The effect of topical amphotericin B on inflammatory markers in patients with chronic rhinosinusitis: a multicenter ran- domized controlled study. Laryngoscope 2009;119(2):401–8.

18. Liang KL, Su MC, Shiao JY, et al. Amphotericin B irrigation for the treatment of chronic rhinosinusitis without nasal polyps: a randomized, placebo-controlled, double-blind study. Am J Rhinol 2008;22(1):52–8.

19. Leopold DA, Elkayam D, Messina JC, et al. NAVIGATE II: Randomized, double- blind trial of the exhalation delivery system with fluticasone for nasal polyposis. J Allergy Clin Immunol 2019;143(1):126–34.e5.

20. Messina JC, Offman E, Carothers JL, et al. A randomized comparison of the phar- macokinetics and bioavailability of fluticasone propionate delivered via xhance exhalation delivery system versus flonase nasal spray and flovent HFA inhala- tional aerosol. Clin Ther 2019;41(11):2343–56.

21. Lavigne F, Miller SK, Gould AR, et al. Steroid-eluting sinus implant for in-office treatment of recurrent nasal polyposis: a prospective, multicenter study. Int Forum Allergy Rhinol 2014;4(5):381–9.

22. Han JK, Forwith KD, Smith TL, et al. RESOLVE: a randomized, controlled, blinded study of bioabsorbable steroid-eluting sinus implants for in-office treatment of recurrent sinonasal polyposis. Int Forum Allergy Rhinol 2014;4(11):861–70.

23. Rivero A, Liang J. Anti-IgE and anti-IL5 biologic therapy in the treatment of nasal polyposis: a systematic review and meta-analysis. Ann Otol Rhinol Laryngol 2017;126(11):739–47.

24. Yamada T, Fujieda S, Mori S, et al. Macrolide treatment decreased the size of nasal polyps and IL-8 levels in nasal lavage. Am J Rhinol 2000;14(3):143–8.

25. Scangas GA, Remenschneider AK, Su BM, et al. Cost utility analysis of endoscopic sinus surgery for chronic rhinosinusitis with and without nasal polyposis. Laryngoscope 2017;127(1):29–37.

26. Smith KA, Orlandi RR, Oakley G, et al. Long-term revision rates for endoscopic sinus surgery. Int Forum Allergy Rhinol 2019;9(4):402–8.

27. Snidvongs K, Pratt E, Chin D, et al. Corticosteroid nasal irrigations after endoscopic sinus surgery in the management of chronic rhinosinusitis. Int Forum Allergy Rhinol 2012;2(5):415–21.

28. Yoo F, Ference EH, Kuan EC, et al. Evaluation of patient nasal saline irrigation practices following endoscopic sinus surgery. Int Forum Allergy Rhinol 2018; 8(1):32–40.

Otorhinolaryngology Manifestations of Systemic Illness

Esther Lee III, BS[a,b,*], Christopher Badger, MD[a],
Punam G. Thakkar, MD[a]

KEYWORDS

- Otorhinolaryngology • ENT • Systemic disease

KEY POINTS

- Ear-nose-throat (ENT) manifestations are among the most frequently observed clinical features of systemic illnesses, and physicians should have a high index of suspicion to identify the underlying disease.
- ENT manifestations that are commonly encountered include lobular capillary hemangioma, systemic lupus erythematosus, rheumatoid arthritis, Sjögren syndrome, relapsing polychondritis, granulomatosis with polyangiitis, Behçet disease, Cogan syndrome, sarcoidosis, human immunodeficiency virus, and oral candidiasis.
- Early recognition and prompt treatment or referral to specialists may prevent morbidity and mortality related to systemic diseases.

INTRODUCTION

Ear-nose-throat (ENT) manifestations are among the most frequently observed clinical features of systemic illnesses.[1] The patients often present with overt findings of head and neck lesions, such as salivary gland swelling or lymphadenopathy, that appear as early as the patients can notice. In contrast, the patients may present with covert findings of auditory, nasal, and laryngeal symptoms that are less obvious and can often be overlooked. Therefore, clinicians should have a high index of suspicion to identify the underlying disease because undiagnosed systemic illness often requires an immediate and chronic immunosuppressive treatment. Early recognition and prompt treatment or referral to specialists may prevent morbidity and mortality related to these diseases. This article presents various systemic illnesses with ENT manifestations

[a] Division of Otolaryngology–Head and Neck Surgery, George Washington University School of Medicine & Health Sciences, 2300 M Street Northwest 4th Floor, Washington, DC 20037, USA;
[b] Western University of Health Sciences, 309 E. Second Street, Pomona, CA 91766, USA
* Corresponding author. Division of Otolaryngology–Head and Neck Surgery, George Washington University School of Medicine & Health Sciences, 2300 M Street Northwest 4th Floor, Washington, DC 20037.
E-mail address: estlee@mfa.gwu.edu

Med Clin N Am 105 (2021) 871–883
https://doi.org/10.1016/j.mcna.2021.05.009
0025-7125/21/© 2021 Elsevier Inc. All rights reserved.

that are commonly encountered, including lobular capillary hemangioma (LCH), systemic lupus erythematosus (SLE), rheumatoid arthritis (RA), Sjögren syndrome (SS), relapsing polychondritis (RP), Behçet disease, Cogan syndrome, sarcoidosis, human immunodeficiency virus (HIV), and oral candidiasis (OC).

DISCUSSION
Lobular Capillary Hemangioma (Pyogenic Granuloma)

LCH may occur throughout the body, but head and neck manifestations are usually associated with the mucosa of the upper airway. Mucosal LCH presents as a rapidly growing nodule or papule of the upper airway mucosa that is typically painless. It usually manifests as a red-purple papule or nodule ranging in size from a few millimeters to 2.5 cm. Lesions may be sessile or pedunculated[2] and bleed with minor trauma (**Fig. 1**). LCH of the head and neck is most commonly found in the oral cavity, such as on the lip or gingival mucosa,[3] but may also affect the nasal cavity. When found in the nasal cavity, it is frequently associated with epistaxis (75%) or nasal obstruction (36%).[4] Although historically called a pyogenic granuloma, LCH does not represent infection nor is it a true granuloma. LCH is theorized to be a hyperplastic, neovascular response to angiogenic stimulation such as trauma or hormonal promotion. Lesions may affect all ages, but intraoral LCH is regularly seen during the first 5 months of pregnancy (3%) and typically resolves spontaneously after childbirth.[2] Most cases of mucosal LCH are treated with surgical excision to avoid the repeated bleeding and ulceration frequently associated with such lesions.

Systemic Lupus Erythematosus

There are 3 subtypes of lupus: discoid lupus erythematosus, subacute cutaneous lupus, and SLE. Among these, SLE represents the most severe form, with a wide range of systemic manifestations. Oral lesions can be seen in approximately 25% of patients with SLE. Oral lesions are often located on the lips and mucosal surfaces, where they usually present as superficial ulcers with surrounding erythema.[5] Other oral

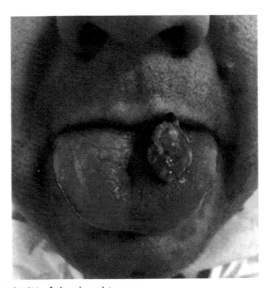

Fig. 1. Pedunculated LCH of the dorsal tongue.

manifestations of SLE include periodontal diseases, xerostomia, and hyposalivation, which can occur with or without SS.[6] SLE may also present with nasal manifestations. However, nasal mucosal involvement in SLE is an under-researched area and its prevalence is not clearly documented, because most studies combine the prevalence of oral and nasal ulcers. A long list of nasal manifestations is documented in the literature, which includes nasal congestion, epistaxis, nasal crusting, rhinorrhea, nasal ulcers, and septal perforation.[7] Of all the nasal manifestations, only nasal ulcer is part of the clinical Systemic Lupus International Collaborating Clinics criteria.[8]

Diagnosis is established with direct and indirect immunofluorescence of the oral lesion staining the basement membrane of the dermal-epidermal junction with immunoglobulins and complement. The microscopic diagnosis is critical because oral lesions from SLE are often clinically indistinguishable from lichen planus and leukoplakia.[9] Blood studies should also include antinuclear and anti–double-stranded DNA antibodies.

Rheumatoid Arthritis

RA is one of the most prevalent chronic inflammatory diseases, affecting approximately 1% of the population worldwide.[10] RA primarily affects the joints of the hands, wrists, elbows, shoulders, hips, knees, and feet, but less frequently involves other joints, such as the temporomandibular joints (TMJs). More than half of patients with RA clinically show TMJ involvement.[11] Symptoms of TMJ include clicking, locking, crepitus, tenderness in the preauricular area, and pain during masseteric muscle contraction.[12] In advanced stages, TMJ may present with malocclusion of the teeth and anterior open bite.[13] Although the findings of TMJ on radiographs vary, the main changes are flattening, spiked deformity, or a pencil-like condylar head, and cortical erosion.[14] Initial management of arthritic-associated TMJ symptoms is conservative and includes soft diets, antiinflammatory medications, and warm compresses. However, persistent symptoms may benefit from intraoral orthotic devices, physical therapy, and ultimately surgery.

Sjögren Syndrome

RA is also frequently associated with other autoimmune connective tissue diseases, such as SS,[15] which is characterized by sicca complex consisting of xerostomia and xerophthalmia. It is a chronic autoimmune disorder characterized on histopathology by lymphocytic infiltration and destruction of the lacrimal and salivary glands. Up to 50% of patients with primary SS are found to have systemic manifestations in the form of dermatologic, pulmonary, gastroenterologic, renal, neurologic, and hematologic involvement. On head and neck examination, patients may show caries, a hyperlobulated tongue, decreased salivary pooling in the floor of mouth, and a loss of filiform papillae. Systemic findings associated with SS include palpable purpura of the lower extremities, peripheral neuropathy, and OC. This condition can consequently lead to difficulty in swallowing and phonation, sensation of burning mouth, increased thirst, loss of taste, unpleasant taste and odor, and dental sensitivity.[16]

The diagnosis of primary SS is based on the 2016 American College of Rheumatology (ACR) and European League Against Rheumatism (EULAR) classification criteria, a weighted scoring method that includes labial salivary gland biopsy histopathology, serology, abnormal ocular staining scores, Shirmer test, and the unstimulated salivary flow rate.[17] Salivary gland ultrasonography (SGUS) is useful in characterizing primary SS, where it was found to increase diagnostic accuracy when included in existing criteria.[18] SGUS evaluation and scoring systems of the submandibular and parotid glands are based on parenchymal echogenicity, heterogeneity, the presence of hypoechogenic areas, hyperechogenic reflections, and clearness of the salivary gland border (**Fig. 2**).[19] SGUS has been shown to have a high diagnostic accuracy (sensitivity 87.1%, specificity 90.8%), second only to labial minor salivary gland biopsy (91%–94%).[20]

Relapsing Polychondritis

RP is a rare autoimmune disorder of proteoglycan-rich structures and cartilaginous tissues, most often found in auricular pinna, cartilage of the nose, tracheobronchial tree, eyes, and the heart's connective components.[21] RP manifests as sudden onset, with auricular chondritis as the most common manifestation, followed by nasal chondritis, which is found in 24% of patients.[21]

Diagnosis of RP is mainly based on typical clinical findings as well as radiologic imaging tools such as computed tomography and MRI. Treatment is empirically tailored according to disease severity and the nature of organ involvement. Mild symptoms are managed with nonsteroid antiinflammatory drugs, dapsone, or colchicine, whereas the most severe cases are managed with high-dose corticosteroids.[21] Immunosuppressant agents such as azathioprine, methotrexate, and cyclosporine may be administered in unresponsive patients or when a corticosteroid-sparing effect is needed.[17]

Granulomatosis with Polyangiitis (Wegner Granulomatosis)

Granulomatosis with polyangiitis (GPA), formerly known as Wegener granulomatosis, is a systemic necrotizing vasculitis of small and medium-sized blood vessels. GPA commonly occurs in patients aged between 45 and 60 years of both genders.[18] According to the criteria of the ACR, GPA is defined by presence of at least 2 of the following 4 criteria: (1) sinus involvement; (2) lung radiograph showing nodules, a fixed pulmonary infiltrates, or cavities; (3) urinary sediment with hematuria or red cell casts; and (4) histologic granulomas within an artery or a perivascular area of an artery or arteriole.[19]

ENT symptoms are present in 70% to 100% of GPA cases. Nasal-sinus involvement is the most common hallmark of GPA, and nasal obstruction with hyposmia or anosmia is often the presenting symptom.[18] Nasal-sinus manifestations include crusting rhinorrhea; sinusitis; chronic otitis media; damage of the facial cartilage causing saddle nose; and perforation of the nasal septum, palate, or pinna of the ear.[20] Necrotizing granulomas can also develop within the middle ear and mastoid, compromising the ossicular chain and eustachian tube function and resulting in a conductive hearing

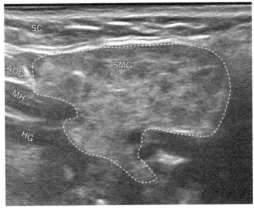

Fig. 2. Submandibular gland (SMG) in a patient with SS. ADG, anterior belly digastric muscle; HG, hyoglossus; MH, mylohyoid, SC, subcutaneous fat, SMG, submandibular gland.

loss.[22] This condition can also develop sensorineural hearing loss, most likely with an autoimmune cause.[22]

The initial treatment is to induce remission with cyclophosphamide (2 mg/kg/d) and high-dose glucocorticoids (prednisone 0.5–1 mg/kg/d). Cyclophosphamide is continued for 6 to 12 months until symptoms disappear and then switched to a less toxic immunosuppressant, such as methotrexate or azathioprine. Steroids are used for 1 month and are slowly tapered over several months.[23]

Behçet Disease

Behçet disease is a multisystem autoimmune condition well known to involve a classic triad of symptoms: recurrent aphthous ulcers, genital ulcers, and uveitis.[24] The highest prevalence of Behçet disease is seen in the Mediterranean, Middle East, and Far East, primarily affecting young people ranging from 20 to 35 years of age.[25]

Recurrent oral ulceration is the most common initial symptom of Behçet disease. The ulcers classically present as multiple, painful, variable-sized (2–20 mm) ulcers that occur on the buccal membrane, tongue, palate, and oropharynx. During the relapse, the oral ulcers become more persistent, lasting up to 6 weeks.[25]

The otologic manifestations of Behçet disease can be divided into sensorineural hearing loss and disequilibrium. The sensorineural hearing loss is variable, with descriptions ranging from unilateral to bilateral, mild to profound, and low-frequency dominant to high-frequency dominant.[25]

The diagnosis of Behçet disease is entirely based on clinical presentations, with a thorough history, physical examination, and exclusion of other autoimmune conditions. Biopsy of oral ulceration is not diagnostic because the ulcers cannot be distinguished from aphthous ulceration.[26] Pure tone audiometry may be helpful for the patients presenting with vertigo.

The treatment of Behçet disease depends on the severity and clinical presentations. Oral ulcerations respond well to topical treatment with tetra-triamcinolone mouthwash.[25] Serious acute episodes can be managed with a short-term course of systemic corticosteroids, as well as immunosuppressants such as azathioprine, cyclosporine, tacrolimus, and mycophenolate motefil.[25] Anti–tumor necrosis factor alpha agents such as infliximab, used to treat RA, have also been shown to be highly effective for Behçet disease.[25] These drugs can be used to treat serious organ involvement when other agents have failed.

Cogan Syndrome

Cogan's syndrome is a rare autoimmune systemic vasculitis characterized by intraocular inflammation and vestibuloauditory dysfunction, sometimes with systemic manifestations. Because no serologic marker for the disease has been found, the diagnosis should be suspected whenever there are ocular abnormalities closely followed or preceded by audiovestibular symptoms.[27] The onset of the disease is preceded by an upper respiratory tract infection in approximately 27% of cases, or by diarrhea, dental infection, or immunization.[28] The ocular manifestation commonly includes interstitial keratitis but can also present with scleritis, episcleritis, retinal vascular disease, uveitis, iritis, conjunctivitis, papilledema, exophthalmos, or tendonitis.[29] The audiovestibular manifestations are very similar to those of Meniere disease, including vertigo, tinnitus, and sensorineural hearing loss, leading to deafness in a period of 1 to 3 months.[30] Physical examination can show ataxia and spontaneous nystagmus. Audiometry examination shows sensorineural hearing loss affecting all frequencies.[31] Auditory evoked potential is also reduced or absent and the caloric test is absent in 70% of patients.[27]

Treatment depends on the severity and the extent of the disease. Interstitial keratitis responds well to corticosteroid eye drops or local atropine. Audiovestibular involvement benefits from early treatment with systemic corticosteroid (eg, 1–2 mg/kg/d prednisolone).[31] If the response to therapy is incomplete, an immunosuppressive agent such as azathioprine, cyclosporine A, methotrexate, or TNF-alpha blockers can be added.[31]

SARCOIDOSIS

Sarcoidosis is a chronic granulomatous disease of multiorgan systems. Diagnosis of sarcoidosis must meet 3 criteria: (1) compatible clinical and radiologic findings, (2) histologic findings of noncaseating granulomas, and (3) exclusion of other granulomatous diseases.[32]

Although sarcoidosis most commonly presents with pulmonary findings, being present in more than 90% of patients, otolaryngologic manifestations are found in 10% to 15% of patients.[32] Cervical adenopathy is the most common head and neck manifestation of sarcoidosis, found in 48% of patients.[33] The diagnosis can be confirmed with ultrasonography-guided fine-needle aspiration or open biopsy.[34] Parotid gland involvement occurs in 6% of patients and may present as Heerfordt disease with parotitis uveitis, facial paralysis, and fever. Biopsy of the affected salivary glands confirms the diagnosis.[35]

Sinonasal manifestations are found in 1% to 4% of patients with sarcoidosis. Typical symptoms include nasal obstruction, postnasal drip, headache, and recurrent sinus infection. Granulomatous infiltrations can result in yellowish nodules. Polypoid tissue and septal perforations can occur, and may lead to saddle nose deformity in severe cases.[36]

Otologic manifestations are rare and may mimic several other diseases of the ear. Sarcoidosis can present as raised, nodular skin lesions on the auricular helix.[35] Middle ear involvement can present with nonspecific symptoms, including otalgia, hearing loss, aural fullness, tinnitus, disequilibrium, and vertigo.[35] Sarcoidosis can, in rare cases, affect the vestibuloacoustic system, which warrants further evaluations, including audiogram, electroneuronography, and MRI.

Laryngeal manifestations are found in 0.5% to 8.3% of patients and may occur in the absence of other manifestations of the disease.[36] It commonly presents in supraglottic structures of the epiglottis, aryepiglottic folds, arytenoids, and false vocal folds, with sparing of the true vocal folds. Laryngeal sarcoid is predisposed to these areas given the high concentration of lymphatic channels in these structures. The disease follows a relapsing and remitting course with treatment and includes periods of inflammation followed by resolution and scarring (**Fig. 3**). Laryngeal involvement may initially be benign, but may lead to dysphagia, dyspnea, globus sensation, and voice changes as the disease progresses. Airway obstruction and voice changes can occur, leading to vagal nerve paralysis.

Systemic corticosteroid is the mainstay treatment of sarcoidosis, especially for life-threatening organ or ocular involvement. Topical or inhaled corticosteroids can be used initially in patients with skin, sinonasal, or laryngeal manifestations to reduce complications of systemic steroids. In refractory cases, cytotoxic agents such as methotrexate and azathioprine can be used.[35]

HUMAN IMMUNODEFICIENCY VIRUS

HIV is an RNA retrovirus that compromises the immune system and increases susceptibility to opportunistic infections and malignancy. Up to 80% of patients infected with

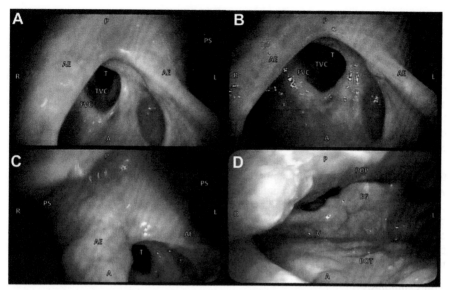

Fig. 3. Laryngeal sarcoidosis. (*A*) Laryngeal sarcoid with prominent supraglottic scarring that spares the true vocal cords (TVC) with extensive scarring of the aryepiglottic (AE) fold and false vocal cords (FVC). (*B, C, D*) Same patient at a different date with inflammation seen in the airway (*B*), edematous nodularity of the AE folds (*C*), and epiglottis (EG) (*D*). A, anterior; BOT, base of tongue; L, left; R, right; P, posterior; POP, posterior oropharyngeal wall; PS, piriform sinus; T, trachea; V, vallecula.

HIV are reported to develop ENT symptoms, with oral manifestations being the most common, followed by neck manifestations.[37] Predisposing factors include cluster of differentiation (CD) cell count of less than 200/μL, plasma HIV-RNA levels greater than 3000 copies/mL, xerostomia, poor oral hygiene, and smoking.[38]

Oral manifestations are the most common symptoms and occur in approximately 40% to 50% of HIV-positive patients.[39] OC, also known as thrush, is the most common oral manifestation and can occur in oropharynx, hypopharynx, and larynx. Mild to moderate symptoms are treated with topical agents such as clotrimazole troches and nystatin oral suspension, and severe symptoms are treated with systemic agents. Oral infections with herpes simplex virus occur in up to 9% of adults with HIV, presenting as a small crop of vesicles on the lips. Although they are typically self-limiting, antiviral agents such as acyclovir can be used.[40] Oral hairy leukoplakia caused by the Epstein-Barr virus presents as a white lesion on the lateral borders of the tongue, and no treatment is required. Oral human papilloma virus infections by subtypes 16 and 18 present as cauliflowerlike lesions and are related to oral sexual behavior. Treatment involves surgical removal, which may need to be repeated because of high recurrence of the lesions.[41] Kaposi sarcoma is the most common oral malignancy in patients infected with HIV. It presents as red to purple lesions that are macular, nodular, or raised. Diagnosis is made with biopsy of the lesion, and it is treated with surgical removal.[40]

Diffuse cervical lymphadenopathy is the most common manifestation of HIV infection in the neck and occurs in up to 70% of patients infected with HIV.[41] It may be the result of reactive lymphadenitis, tuberculosis, lymphoma, or Kaposi sarcoma.[41] The lymph nodes are soft, symmetric, with size range from 1 to 5 cm in diameter, and are most frequently found in the posterior triangle.[42] Diagnosis can be made with fine-needle aspiration and biopsy.

Salivary gland manifestations occur in approximately 3% to 30% of adult patients and most commonly present as a progressive parotid swelling over several months. The 3 common causes of parotid enlargement are hyperplasia of an intraparotid lymph node, benign lymphoepithelial cysts (BLECs) (**Fig. 4**), and benign lymphoepithelial lesions with ductal metaplasia. The diagnosis is made with fine-needle aspiration. The treatment of parotid enlargement remains controversial, ranging from less invasive procedures such as aspiration or doxycycline sclerotherapy, to invasive superficial parotidectomy or external irradiation.[41]

Otologic manifestations in patients with HIV are broad and can involve all 3 parts of the ear. The most common presenting symptom is otalgia from recurrent otitis media, which requires broad-spectrum antibiotics. Sensorineural hearing loss is reported to occur in 21% to 49% of patients infected with HIV from involvement of either retrocochlear pathways or cochlear nerve.[41] Patients with HIV may also experience significant disequilibrium from central nervous system disorder. In addition, facial nerve palsy occurs with 100-fold greater frequency in patients infected with HIV and requires treatment with acyclovir and prednisolone.

Oral Candidiasis

Candida is the normal oral flora of healthy individuals, present in 30% to 55% of healthy adults.[43] There are both systemic and local factors that predispose an overgrowth of *Candida* species in the oral mucosa leading to OC. Systemic factors include immunosuppressed states, such as HIV, leukemia, malnutrition, radiation therapy, chemotherapy, and use of systemic corticosteroid; local factors include use of dentures, corticosteroid inhalers, and xerostomia.[44–46]

There are 4 different forms of OC:

1. Pseudomembranous candidiasis, also known as oral thrush, is the most common type of OC and is commonly found in individuals who are immunosuppressed, such as those taking immunosuppressive medications, using corticosteroid inhalers, developing malignancies, or having immune diseases such as HIV (**Fig. 5**).[47] The

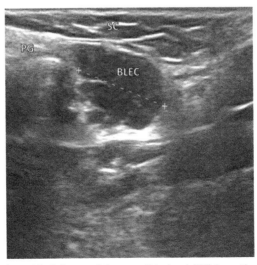

Fig. 4. Benign lymphoepithelial cyst of the parotid gland (PG) in patient with HIV.

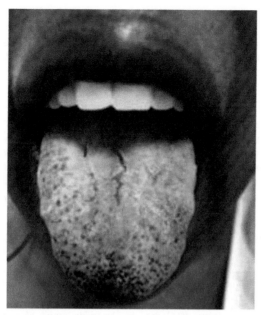

Fig. 5. Pseudomembranous candidiasis (oral thrush) on the tongue.

classic presentation is white curdlike plaques on the tongue, buccal mucosa, hard palate, soft palate, and oral pharynx.[48] White plaques can easily be wiped off with gauze or a tongue blade, leaving behind an erythematous surface.[49]

2. Hyperplastic candidiasis presents as thick white plaques that are commonly adherent to the buccal mucosa.[50] The plaques cannot easily be wiped off, making its distinction from leukoplakia difficult. Hyperplastic candidiasis has also been associated with increased malignant changes compared with noncandidal leukoplakia.[50]

3. Atrophic candidiasis presents as erythematous patches on the palate, buccal mucosa, or dorsal tongue.[51] There may be loss of tongue papillation leading to burning sensation in the mouth and soreness of lip and tongue.[50] It is also known as antibiotic sore mouth because it may occur after use of broad-spectrum antimicrobials, which leads to overgrowth of *Candida albicans*.[47] Other predisposing factors include use of corticosteroids, HIV diseases, uncontrolled diabetes mellitus, iron deficiency anemia, and vitamin B_{12} deficiency.[52–55]

4. Angular cheilitis presents as erythematous cracking and fissuring along the oral commissure. The patients typically complain of soreness and pain with fissuring. It is commonly seen in denture users, as well as those who lick their lips and bite the corners of their mouth.[55] Other predisposing factors include vitamin deficiency of folic acid, iron, riboflavin, thiamine, and vitamin B_{12}.[56]

A diagnosis of OC includes a thorough medical history and physical examination. The diagnosis can be confirmed by a periodic acid–Schiff stain that reveals *Candida* hyphae, or by potassium hydroxide (KOH) that reveals pseudohyphal elements and budding yeast.[47]

For mild cases of OC, topical antifungal agents may be sufficient. However, systemic antifungal therapy is used for disease that is resistant to topical medications or patients at risk for disseminated candidiasis.[47] For OC in patients with HIV, treatment can be managed based on CD4 counts. For CD4 counts greater than 200, topical antifungals such as nystatin mouthwash can be used. For CD4 counts less than 200, systemic antifungals such as fluconazole can be used. Patients with HIV are also at risk of developing fluconazole-resistant *Candida* from repeated treatments.[47]

SUMMARY

Many systemic illnesses manifest in the head, neck, ear, nose, and throat examination because of the large number of physiologic systems involved. It serves as a nexus for most organ systems. Careful and thorough physical examination may guide differential diagnosis and treatment of many systemic illnesses. Early recognition and prompt treatment or referral to the appropriate specialist based on the findings in this examination may prevent morbidity and mortality related to the systemic diseases mentioned and many more.

CLINICS CARE POINTS

- Lobular capillary hemangiomas involving the upper airway can cause life-threatening airway compromise and may require emergent airway management.

- Systemic lupus erythematosus (SLE) may involve wide range of nasal manifestations including nasal ulcer, nasal congestion, and epistaxis. However, nasal mucosa involvement in SLE is under-researched area and are often overlooked.

- Rheumatoid arthritis may less frequently involve temporomandibular joints and can be managed conservatively with soft diets, warm compresses, and anti-inflammatory medications.

- Sjögren's syndrome (SS) presents with characteristic sicca complex consisting of xerostomia and ophthalmia which can be managed conservatively. Systemic symptoms of SS may lead to difficulty in swallowing and phonation, sensation of burning mouth, and more.

- Relapsing polychondritis most commonly involve auricular pinna and cartilage of nose. Treatment is tailored according to disease severity with nonsteroid anti-inflammatory drugs and corticosteroids.

- Granulomatosis with polyangiitis (GPA) often initially present with nasal-sinus manifestations including nasal obstruction, hyposmia, or anosmia. The initial treatment involves cyclophosphamide and high-dose glucocorticoids.

- Behcet's disease often initially present with recurrent painful oral ulceration which responds well to tetra-triamcinolone mouth wash.

- Cogan's syndrome is characterized by vestibulo-auditory dysfunction that present very similarly with Meniere's disease including vertigo, tinnitus, and sensorineural hearing loss. Thorough ocular examination is warranted to diagnosis Cogan's syndrome.

- Sarcoidosis may commonly present with cervical adenopathy and parotid gland involvement. Diagnosis can be confirmed with ultrasound-guided fine needle aspiration.

- Human immunodeficiency virus (HIV) commonly presents with oral candidiasis and are treated with topical antifungal agents.

- Up to 70% of HIV infected patients presents with diffuse cervical lymphadenopathy and fine needle aspiration or biopsy can be use do to exclude malignancy.

DISCLOSURE

The authors have no commercial or financial conflicts of interest or funding sources relevant to this article.

REFERENCES

1. Gusmão RJ, Fernandes FL, Guimarães AC, et al. Otorhinolaryngological findings in a group of patients with rheumatic diseases. Rev Bras Reumatol 2014;54(3):172–8.
2. Maymone MBC, Greer RO, Burdine LK, et al. Benign oral mucosal lesions: clinical and pathological findings. J Am Acad Dermatol 2019;81(1):43–56.
3. Mills SE, Cooper PH, Fechner RE. Lobular capillary hemangioma: the underlying lesion of pyogenic granuloma. A study of 73 cases from the oral and nasal mucous membranes. Am J Surg Pathol 1980;4(5):470–9.
4. Smith SC, Patel RM, Lucas DR, et al. Sinonasal lobular capillary hemangioma: a clinicopathologic study of 34 cases characterizing potential for local recurrence. Head Neck Pathol 2013;7(2):129–34.
5. Freites-Martinez A, Aguado-Lobo M, Calderón-Komaromy A, et al. Mucocutaneous presentation of systemic lupus erythematosus. J Pediatr 2014;165(3):631.
6. Said-Al-Naief N, Rosebush MS, Lynch D. Clinical-pathological conference: case 2. Head Neck Pathol 2010;4(3):221–5.
7. Kusyairi KA, Gendeh BS, Sakthiswary R, et al. The spectrum of nasal involvement in systemic lupus erythematosus and its association with the disease activity. Lupus 2016;25(5):520–4.
8. Petri M, Orbai A-M, Alarcón GS, et al. Derivation and validation of the systemic lupus international collaborating clinics classification criteria for systemic lupus erythematosus. Arthritis Rheum 2012;64(8):2677–86.
9. Cummings C, Flint P. Cummings otolaryngology - head & neck surgery. St. Louis: Mosby Elsevier; 2020.
10. Gibofsky A. Epidemiology, pathophysiology, and diagnosis of rheumatoid arthritis: a synopsis. Am J Manag Care 2014;20(7 Suppl):S128–35.
11. Sodhi A, Naik S, Pai A, et al. Rheumatoid arthritis affecting temporomandibular joint. Contemp Clin Dent 2015;6(1):124–7.
12. Yıldırım D, Türkkahraman H, Yılmaz HH, et al. Dentofacial characteristics of patients with rheumatoid arthritis. Clin Oral Investig 2013;17(7):1677–83.
13. Scutellari PN, Orzincolo C. Rheumatoid arthritis: sequences. Eur J Radiol 1998;27:S31–8.
14. Goupille P, Fouquet B, Cotty P, et al. Direct coronal computed tomography of the temporomandibular joint in patients with rheumatoid arthritis. Br J Radiol 1992;65(779):955–60.
15. Flint PW, Haughey BH, Robbins KT, et al. Cummings otolaryngology - head and neck surgery E-book. 6th ed. Saunders; 2014.
16. Chamani G, Shakibi MR, Zarei MR, et al. Assessment of relationship between xerostomia and oral health-related quality of life in patients with rheumatoid arthritis. Oral Dis 2017;23(8):1162–7.
17. Sharma A, Gnanapandithan K, Sharma K, et al. Relapsing polychondritis: a review. Clin Rheumatol 2013;32(11):1575–83.
18. Comarmond C, Cacoub P. Granulomatosis with polyangiitis (Wegener): clinical aspects and treatment. Autoimmun Rev 2014;13(11):1121–5.

19. Leavitt RY, Fauci AS, Bloch DA, et al. The American College of Rheumatology 1990 criteria for the classification of Wegener's granulomatosis. Arthritis Rheum 1990;33:1101–7.

20. Trimarchi M, Sinico RA, Teggi R, et al. Otorhinolaryngological manifestations in granulomatosis with polyangiitis (Wegener's). Autoimmun Rev 2013;12(4):501–5.

21. Vitale A, Sota J, Rigante D, et al. Relapsing polychondritis: an update on pathogenesis, clinical features, diagnostic tools, and therapeutic perspectives. Curr Rheumatol Rep 2016;18(1):3.

22. Themes UFO. Otologic manifestations of systemic disease: includes autoimmune inner ear disease. 2016. Available at: https://entokey.com/otologic-manifestations-of-systemic-disease-includes-autoimmune-inner-ear-disease/. Accessed October 28, 2020.

23. Chapter 13. Nasal manifestations of systemic disease. Available at: https://accessmedicine.mhmedical.com/content.aspx?bookid=386&sectionid=39944046. Accessed November 12, 2020.

24. Shahram F, Assadi K, Davatchi F, et al. Chronology of clinical manifestations in Behçet's disease. Analysis of 4024 cases. Adv Exp Med Biol 2003;528:85–9.

25. Webb CJ, Moots RJ, Swift AC. Ear, nose and throat manifestations of Behçet's disease: a review. J Laryngol Otol 2008;122(12):1279–83.

26. Rhee S-H, Kim Y-B, Lee E-S. Comparison of behçet's disease and recurrent aphthous ulcer according to characteristics of gastrointestinal symptoms. J Korean Med Sci 2005;20(6):971–6.

27. Iliescu DA, Timaru CM, Batras M, et al. Cogan's syndrome. Rom J Ophthalmol 2015;59(1):6–13.

28. Grasland A, Pouchot J, Hachulla E, et al. Typical and atypical Cogan's syndrome: 32 cases and review of the literature. Rheumatology (Oxford) 2004;43(8):1007–15.

29. Berrocal JRG, Vargas JA, Vaquero M, et al. Eponyms in medicine revisited: Cogan's syndrome: an oculo-audiovestibular disease. Postgrad Med J 1999;75(883):262–4.

30. Belhoucha B, Belghmidi S. Atypical cogan's syndrome: case report of an oculoaudiovestibular disease. Am J Med Case Rep 2014;2:139–42.

31. Gaubitz M, Lübben B, Seidel M, et al. Cogan's syndrome: organ-specific autoimmune disease or systemic vasculitis? A report of two cases and review of the literature. Clin Exp Rheumatol 2001;19(4):463–9.

32. Badhey AK, Kadakia S, Carrau RL, et al. Sarcoidosis of the head and neck. Head Neck Pathol 2015;9(2):260–8.

33. Dash GI, Kimmelman CP. Head and neck manifestations of sarcoidosis. Laryngoscope 1988;98(1):50–3.

34. Frable MA, WJ Frable. Fine needle aspiration biopsy in the diagnosis of sarcoid of the head and neck.

35. Schwartzbauer HR, Tami TA. Ear, nose, and throat manifestations of sarcoidosis. Otolaryngol Clin North Am 2003;36(4):673–84.

36. Gallivan GJ, JN Landis. Sarcoidosis of the larynx: preserving and restoring airway and professional voice.

37. Sanjar FA, Queiroz BEUP, Miziara ID. Otolaryngologic manifestations in HIV disease–clinical aspects and treatment. Braz J Otorhinolaryngol 2011;77(3):391–400.

38. Tappuni AR, Fleming GJ. The effect of antiretroviral therapy on the prevalence of oral manifestations in HIV-infected patients: a UK study. Oral Surg Oral Med Oral Pathol Oral Radiol Endod 2001;92(6):623–8.

39. Johnson NW, Glick M, Mbuguye TNL. (A2) Oral health and general health. Adv Dent Res 2006;19(1):118–21.
40. Available at: https://www.clinicalkey.com/#!/content/playContent/1-s2.0-S1808869415308715?returnurl=https://linkinghub.elsevier.com/retrieve/pii/S1808869415308715?showall=true&referrer=https://pubmed.ncbi.nlm.nih.gov/. Accessed November 12, 2020.
41. Iacovou E, Vlastarakos PV, Papacharalampous G, et al. Diagnosis and treatment of HIV-associated manifestations in otolaryngology. Infect Dis Rep 2012;4(1):e9.
42. Prasad HKC, Bhojwani KM, Shenoy V, et al. HIV manifestations in otolaryngology. Am J Otolaryngol 2006;27(3):179–85.
43. Arendorf TM, Walker DM. The prevalence and intra-oral distribution of Candida albicans in man. Arch Oral Biol 1980;25(1):1–10.
44. Gonsalves WC, Chi AC, Neville WB. Common oral lesions: part I. *Superficial mucosal lesions*. Am Fam Physician 2007;75:501–7.
45. Fotos PG, Vincent SD, Hellstein JW. Oral candidiasis. Clinical, historical, and therapeutic features of 100 cases. Oral Surg Oral Med Oral Pathol 1992;74:41–9.
46. Abu-Elteen KH, Abu-Alteen RM. The prevalence of Candida albicans populations in the mouths of complete denture wearers. New Microbiol 1998;21:41–8.
47. Millsop JW, Fazel N. Oral candidiasis. Clin Dermatol 2016;34(4):487–94.
48. Sharon V, Fazel N. Oral candidiasis and angular cheilitis. Dermatol Ther 2010;23:230–42.
49. Farah CS, Lynch N, McCullough JM. Oral fungal infections: an update for the general practitioner. Aust Dent J 2010;55(Suppl. 1):48–54.
50. Akpan A. Oral candidiasis. Postgrad Med J 2002;78(922):455–9.
51. McCullough MJ, Savage WN. Oral candidiasis and the therapeutic use of antifungal agents in dentistry. Aust Dent J 2005;50:36–9.
52. Ellepola AN, Samaranayake PL. Inhalational and topical steroids, and oral candidiasis: a mini review. Oral Dis 2001;7:211.
53. Giannini PJ, Shetty VK. Diagnosis and management of oral candidiasis Otolaryngol. Clin North Am 2011;44:231–40.
54. Ramirez-Amador V, Esquivel-Pedraza L, Sierra-Madero J, et al. Oral manifestations of HIV infection by gender and transmission category in Mexico City. J Oral Pathol Med 1998;27(3):135–40.
55. Appleton SS. Candidiasis: pathogenesis, clinical characteristics, and treatment. J Calif Dent Assoc 2000;28:942–8.
56. Rose AJ. Folic-acid deficiency as a cause of angular cheilosis. Lancet 1971;2:453–4.

Obstructive Sleep Apnea
A Surgeon's Perspective

Kara D. Brodie, MD, MPhil, Andrew N. Goldberg, MD, MSCE*

KEYWORDS

- Obstructive sleep apnea • Otolaryngology • Sleep medicine • Sleep surgery

KEY POINTS

- Obstructive sleep apnea (OSA) is a complex medical disorder with significant impact on mortality, quality of life, and long-term cardiovascular outcomes.
- Surgical intervention should be considered in patients who are noncompliant with or fail continuous positive airway pressure use.
- Improvement in OSA from surgery does not rely on patient compliance; therefore, patients benefit each night.
- Surgery improves mortality and symptoms of OSA even when the polysomnogram does not normalize.
- Although the apnea-hypopnea index has been used to quantify severity of disease and treatment success, it does not correlate well with either quality-of-life measures or health outcomes such as hypertension. Therefore, response to treatment should incorporate other metrics as well.

FRAMING THE PROBLEM OF OBSTRUCTIVE SLEEP APNEA
Background

Obstructive sleep apnea (OSA) is the symptomatic, repeated upper airway obstruction occurring during sleep, resulting in reduced or complete cessation of airflow.[1] OSA affects 3% to 9% of men and 2% to 5% of women in the United States, in total about 18 million to 20 million American adults.[2–4] Obesity, male gender, and age are all independent risk factors, with obesity having the strongest association with OSA. Individuals with OSA may endorse poor sleep quality, daytime somnolence, reduced cognition, and morning headaches.

There are significant differences in the epidemiology, pathophysiology, and management of pediatric OSA. This article focuses on OSA as it pertains to the adult population.

Division of Rhinology and Sinus Surgery, Department of Otolaryngology, Head and Neck Surgery, University of California, San Francisco, 2233 Post Street, Room 309, San Francisco, CA 94115-1225, USA
* Corresponding author.
E-mail address: Andrew.Goldberg@ucsf.edu

Med Clin N Am 105 (2021) 885–900
https://doi.org/10.1016/j.mcna.2021.05.010
medical.theclinics.com

Pathophysiology

The underlying pathophysiology of OSA is complex and varies across individuals. Upper airway collapse and consequent airway obstruction in OSA is caused by the combination of predisposing upper airway anatomy and decreased muscle tone while sleeping. Obstruction can be accentuated during rapid eye movement (REM) sleep, when significant muscle hypotonia occurs.[1] Oropharyngeal, hypopharyngeal, or epiglottic obstruction results in intermittent hypercapnia and hypoxemia, causing increases in sympathetic stimulation and nighttime arousals. Anatomic soft tissue variations that can create obstruction in the oropharynx include enlarged tonsils, long uvula, excessive pharyngeal mucosal folds, webbing of posterior tonsillar pillars, and low-lying soft palate. Bony anatomy, particularly retrognathia of the mandible, can also predispose to a narrow airway and subsequent OSA. Hypopharyngeal anatomic variants such as an enlarged base of tongue, lingual tonsillar hypertrophy, and an enlarged, collapsed, or prolapsing epiglottis can cause obstruction. Studies have found that a genetic predisposition for OSA exists, such as an association with a narrow oropharynx.[5–7] Men are more likely to develop OSA than women, possibly because of thickened musculature, higher pharyngeal fat deposition, and increased pharyngeal length; however, the basis is not well elucidated.[1]

Nasal obstruction has significant implications in OSA, affecting about 45% of patients with OSA.[8] Nasal obstruction can precipitate upper airway collapse because of the increased inspiratory pressure necessary for airflow and subsequently precipitates collapse. This nasal airway resistance accounts for approximately two-thirds of upper airway resistance and is exacerbated by a deviated septum, inferior turbinate hypertrophy, internal or external nasal collapse, or polyps. Because resistance is proportional to the radius of the nasal passageway to the fourth power, small increases in nasal cavity radius have a significant impact on overall airway resistance. Allergic rhinitis alone has been shown to nearly double the risk of having sleep disordered breathing.[9]

Disease Description

Although OSA commonly presents with daytime somnolence, fatigue, and poor sleep quality, these symptoms can be associated with a wide variety of conditions. Therefore, it is imperative to screen for other causes of sleep disturbance, such as depression, anxiety, insomnia, narcolepsy, restless leg syndrome, REM sleep behavior disorder, and central sleep apnea. Furthermore, there are many other conditions that can cause fatigue, including cancer, anemia, autoimmune conditions, renal or hepatic insufficiency, and endocrine abnormalities (diabetes, hypercalcemia, adrenal, and thyroid insufficiency), which should be evaluated in the initial work-up for fatigue.[10] Timeline of symptoms, timing of sleep disturbances, and corroboration from sleeping partners can help to differentiate these conditions. Patients with OSA often deny difficulty falling asleep, but note restless, interrupted, or poor quality sleep. Sleeping partners often endorse loud snoring with intermittent choking sounds that prompt nighttime awakening.

Evaluation for OSA is critical not only for diagnosis but also for prognostication and treatment options. Although there are key presenting signs and symptoms that raise concern for OSA, the diagnosis is typically confirmed by polysomnography.

Disease Assessment: What Is Being Treated?

Research over the last 25 years has consistently shown that apnea-hypopnea index (AHI) does not correlate well with severity of anatomic obstruction, patient perception of disease severity, symptoms of OSA, quality of life, or survival.[11–14] Therefore, targeting AHI alone as the measurement of treatment response does not necessarily result in improved morbidity, mortality, or quality of life. A large proportion of the continuous positive airway pressure (CPAP) literature discusses polysomnographic changes in AHI, but does not evaluate CPAP adherence, thereby overestimating the success of CPAP.[15] More recently, sleep medicine, similar to many other medical fields, is recognizing the value and underappreciation for patient-reported outcome measures and quality-of-life metrics in determining treatment success and is finding independent associations of these metrics with morbidity and mortality data. Given the lack of association with the outcomes of interest, many investigators argue that clinicians must instead focus on reducing morbidity and mortality, such as daytime sleepiness, cognitive performance, cardiovascular disease, and sleep deprivation–associated mortality.

Polysomnography

OSA is typically defined by the number and type of obstructions measured on a polysomnogram (PSG) or sleep study.

Portable PSGs, also referred to as home sleep studies, are commonly used for diagnosis. They can measure obstruction and record oxygenation levels; however, they cannot determine sleep time or sleep stage. Consequently, portable PSGs often underestimate the severity of the OSA by averaging oxygenation patterns while awake during the time period in which the study is performed. Overnight oximetry can be used to screen, rather than diagnose, OSA given the high sensitivity of 98%, but specificity is as low as 40%.[16]

When portable PSGs are suspected to be inaccurate, formal in-laboratory sleep PSGs can be performed, which include electroencephalography, electrocardiography, submental electromyography (EMG), anterior tibialis EMG, and electrooculography, and measure nasal/oral airflow, oxygenation level, respiratory effort, and sleeping position, to calculate the sleep stage, AHI, and respiratory disturbance index (RDI). In addition, some PSGs calculate the respiratory effort–related arousals (RERAs).

Although PSGs are the gold standard for diagnosis of OSA, there are limitations. Namely, sleep patterns that occur in a laboratory with all of the monitors do not always reflect an individual's normal sleep pattern. The Centers for Medicaid and Medicare Services have approved portable PSGs, or home sleep studies, to diagnose OSA.

Before clinicians can further assess work-up and management of OSA, they must first define commonly used terms. These terms refer to airflow limitation and oxygen saturation, which are complete (apnea) or partial (hypopnea), as well as arousals (RERAs) related to obstruction and vibration. The definitions on PSG are included in **Table 1**.

The AHI provides the number of combined apneas and hypopneas in 1 hour. Mild, moderate, and severe OSA are defined by an AHI of 5 to 15, greater than 15 to 30, and greater than 30 respectively. The general parlance of mild, moderate, or severe can also be influenced by desaturation. For example, a patient with severe desaturation may be moved from the moderate to the severe category.

In general, the 2 different definitions of hypopneas have strong agreement in AHI.[17] The AASM criteria for hypopnea (ie, a 3% desaturation) tends to result in higher AHIs compared with Medicare, which uses a 4% desaturation criterion for hypopnea. However, this difference is no longer significant in patients more than 65 years of age.[18]

RERAs, include sleep arousals with associated changes in airflow or respiratory effort without meeting criteria for apneas or hypopneas. When RERAs are reported,

Table 1 Defining terms	
Term	Definition
Apnea	Cessation of airflow for $\geq$10 s
Hypopnea	AASM: 40% reduction in airflow with resultant desaturation of $\geq$4% Medicare: 30% decrease in nasal pressure with >3% desaturation
RERA	Reduction in airflow, despite respiratory effort, with resultant arousal but not meeting criteria for hypopnea
AHI	Average total of apneas and hypopneas per hour of sleep
RDI	Average apneas, hypopneas, and RERAs per hour of sleep
OSA	AHI or RDI $\geq$5, of which >50% are obstructive, with associated clinical symptoms
Central sleep apnea	AHI $\geq$5, of which >50% lack respiratory effort, with associated clinical symptoms

Abbreviation: AASM, American Academy of Sleep Medicine.

the RDI can be calculated as the sum of the AHI and RERAs, which has been shown to be an independent predictor of cardiovascular mortality.[19] For patients with borderline AHI, the RDI can help quantify other sleep disturbances.

Quality-of-Life Indicators

Because OSA has a significant impact on quality of life, it is important to assess the impact of the condition, as well as consequent treatment, on the patient's quality of life. Validated patient-completed questionnaires, including the Epworth Sleepiness Scale (ESS), Sleep Apnea Quality of Life Index, Functional Outcomes of Sleep Questionnaire, and the Pittsburgh Sleep Quality Index, are the most commonly used tools in research and clinical practices to assess the impact of OSA on daily life. The ESS is the single most common clinical measure and is discussed throughout the sleep medicine literature. The ESS is a self-administered patient survey of 8 questions regarding likelihood of falling asleep in different scenarios, including reading, watching television, lying down, or sitting in traffic. Scores greater than 10 points are considered abnormal.[20] Self-reported sleepiness in patients with OSA is associated with increased risk of hypertension to a greater degree than AHI, making the assessment of symptoms a critical part of evaluating and treating patients with sleep disordered breathing.[21]

Associated Morbidity and Mortality

Snoring is the most common symptom that brings patients to seek medical attention and can be bothersome to both patients and their sleeping partners. OSA can have dramatic impacts on quality of life caused by chronic sleep disruption and has been found to be associated with many systemic medical conditions, suspected to be caused by increased cortisol stimulation and subsequent sympathetic activity, systemic inflammation, and endothelial dysfunction.[22] OSA is often associated with depression, hypertension, coronary artery disease, arrhythmia, pulmonary hypertension, and polycythemia. Furthermore, OSA has been shown to have lasting impact on endocrine health and is an independent risk factor for myocardial infarction, cerebrovascular events, and motor vehicle collisions.[23]

EVALUATION
Physical Examination

Anatomic variants of the facial structure can lead to upper airway obstruction. Narrowing of the craniofacial structure, such as mandibular retrognathia, or hypertrophy of the soft tissue of the upper airway both lead to obstruction. Effective intervention must be directed at the single or multiple sites of obstruction. The physical examination is essential to identifying pretest probability of OSA as well as areas to target with intervention. It is important to also assess the height, weight, and body mass index (BMI), because obesity can contribute to multilevel obstruction and can influence clinical outcomes. In the physical examination, the following must be assessed:

Overall: body habitus and BMI
Neck: neck circumference measured at the cricoid
Nose: nasal valve collapse, hypertrophic turbinates, deviated septum
Oral cavity/oropharynx/jaw: **Fig. 1** provides an additional grading system
  Uvula normal/long (<1 cm, >1 cm); thick/thin
  Palate thick/thin, posterior/normal (compared with the posterior pharyngeal wall)
  Tongue: normal (at or just above the bite plane)
    Large (significantly above bite plane)
Tonsils: graded 1 to 4+ or surgically absent
  % of pharynx:
    1+: 0% to 25%
    2+: 25% to 50%
    3+: 50% to 75%
    4+: greater than 75%
Jaw: assessment of retrognathia (**Fig. 2**)
Lateral view with the tragus and infraorbital rim in a horizontal plane
Chin >2 mm behind lower lip is suspicious for retrognathia

Neck circumference greater than 15 inches in women and 17 inches in men is predictive of OSA. The tongue is often a large contributor to obstruction. However, it is not only the size but also the position of the tongue. Even small tongues, when displaced posteriorly because of retrognathia, can cause obstruction. Retrognathia is defined as the posterior displacement of the chin.

The patient is visualized in the lateral view with the tragus and infraorbital rim in a horizontal plane. The chin is normally 2 mm behind a vertical line dropped from the lower lip. If the chin is greater than 2 mm behind lower lip, as in **Fig. 2**, this indicates clinical retrognathia.

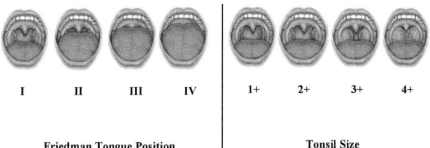

| I | II | III | IV | 1+ | 2+ | 3+ | 4+ |

Friedman Tongue Position   **Tonsil Size**

Fig. 1. Friedman tongue position and tonsil size.

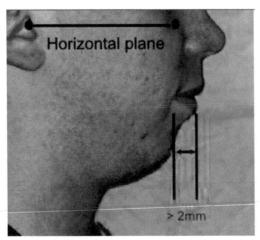

Fig. 2. A simplified method to assess clinical retrognathia.

Friedman Staging System

A standardized method to assess oropharyngeal crowding is the modified Mallampati score, or Friedman tongue position. Crowding of the oropharynx is assessed with the mouth open without protruding the tongue.

The Friedman tongue position and tonsil size (**Fig. 1**) are used in conjunction with the BMI to evaluate candidacy for surgical intervention. The Friedman Staging System (partially shown in **Fig. 1**) uses these 3 measures to guide treatment and predict surgical outcomes.[24]

Flexible Nasopharyngoscopy

In the otolaryngology office, awake flexible nasopharyngoscopy is performed to evaluate the deeper structures of the nasal cavity, nasopharynx, and oropharynx. Specifically, nasopharyngoscopy can assess inferior turbinate hypertrophy, septal deviation, nasal polyps, adenoid hypertrophy, retropalatal narrowing, oropharyngeal width, tonsillar and lateral pharyngeal wall obstruction, tongue base size, lingual hypertrophy, epiglottic malacia, or obstruction to determine whether there are any anatomic variants narrowing the upper airway.

Imaging

At present, imaging, such as computed tomography or MRI, has little clinical utility in diagnosing OSA, related to the static nature and poor predictability of severity or surgical outcomes. However, patients with OSA have been found to have larger tongue volume, lateral pharyngeal wall volume, overall oropharyngeal soft tissue volume, and decreased retropalatal space on cross-sectional imaging.[25,26] Imaging can have a prominent role for evaluating bony structure, particularly of the mandible and maxilla. This imaging is critical for treatment decisions involving surgery of the upper and lower jaws.

Drug-Induced Sleep Endoscopy

Drug-induced sleep endoscopy (DISE) is now a commonly performed dynamic assessment of a patient's upper airway to determine the level of obstruction in a state of drug-induced sleep. The patient is brought to a procedure or operating room where anesthesia can be induced. The patient is induced with a propofol infusion to reproduce the patterns of sleep disordered breathing that occurs during non-REM and REM sleep.[27,28] A flexible nasopharyngoscope is used to visualize airway collapse during carefully titrated sedation in the supine position. A classification system that evaluates the velum, oropharynx, tongue base, and epiglottis provides a structured approach to DISE.[29] Each anatomic segment is graded with regard to level and severity of obstruction.

The benefits of DISE are that it is easy to perform, noninvasive, cost-efficient, and provides a dynamic assessment of patients' obstructive patterns while sleeping. The main disadvantages and risks of DISE include the need for a trained otolaryngologist and anesthesiologist or certified registered nurse anesthetist, the time needed for an accurate assessment, and the risk of respiratory depression if overly sedated.

Multilevel Obstruction

Lee and colleagues[30] performed a recent meta-analysis of 19 studies with 2950 patients and found 57.5% had multilevel obstruction, most commonly involving the soft palate (84%), tongue base (52%), tonsils (33%), and epiglottis (34%). A multi-institutional center study found that oropharyngeal lateral wall collapse during DISE was associated with poorer postsurgical success at 50%.[31] Patients with complete tongue obstruction also had poorer surgical success at 52%. The velum and complete concentric collapse were not as reliable at predicting outcomes.

Treatment Options for Obstructive Sleep Apnea

Patients should be fully informed of the options that are available and then have recommendations personalized based on their level of disease, physical examination, and tolerance. Patients should have a good understanding of the full breadth of nonsurgical treatment options before recommendations for surgery. Any physician treating patients with OSA should perform a physical examination and make appropriate referrals when questions on anatomic obstruction arise. This approach may include referral to an otolaryngologist, oral surgeon, dentist who specializes in oral appliances for sleep, or pulmonologist for optimization of treatment of other sleep disorders or positive airway pressure (PAP) management. Except in certain circumstances (eg, 3–4+ tonsils, significant retrognathia of the mandible), surgery is generally reserved for patients who have inadequate response or poor compliance with nonsurgical interventions.

NONSURGICAL OPTIONS
Behavioral Modifications and Weight Loss

As with most chronic conditions, behavioral modification is the first recommendation in treatment of OSA. Alcohol and sedative sleep aids should be avoided before bedtime, because they increase muscle relaxation and hypotonia and disrupt the natural sleep cycle.

Weight often has a large contribution to OSA, so weight loss is universally recommended. Ten percent weight loss equates to a 26% improvement in AHI.[32] Increasing physical activity to 25 min/d resulted in significant weight loss and AHI reduction, with sustained AHI reduction despite weight gain over time.[33] Overall, about 10% to 20% of patients with OSA can adequately treat their OSA with diet and exercise alone, making this worthwhile for a segment, but not all, of the intended population.[34]

Approximately half of patients have a significant difference in AHI score depending on the sleeping position. Patients can be counseled to sleep in the lateral or prone position, but many need a sleep trainer to assist in maintaining a lateral position. For best effect, padded training belts, foam blocks, electric stimulators, and pillows have been successfully used to promote lateral decubitus sleeping.

Positive Airway Pressure

Continuous PAP (CPAP) is a first-line treatment of OSA and has been shown to reduce somnolence and overall morbidity and mortality in compliant patients. However, about 46% to 83% of patients are noncompliant with CPAP,[35] defined as greater than 4 4h/night on greater than 70% of nights. CPAP units now have the capability of monitoring pressures administered, mask leaks, as well as CPAP usage and adherence to help assess responses and optimize benefit. Barriers to use include claustrophobia, air leak, intolerance of air pressure, epistaxis, equipment failure, social stigma, and failure to address comorbid sleep conditions. CPAP success during titration is generally defined as either reduction of AHI to less than 10 or greater than 75% reduction in AHI.

However, recent randomized trials show that CPAP may not significantly benefit cardiovascular health. A landmark randomized controlled trial found that rates of repeat revascularization, myocardial infarction, stroke, or cardiovascular mortality did not differ significantly in patients who did versus did not receive CPAP, but it did note a significant cardiovascular risk reduction in patients who used CPAP for greater than 4 hours.[36] Studies have shown that patients with OSA treated with CPAP for at least 3 years have lower rates of motor vehicle collisions, comparable with the average population, compared with those with OSA who are not on CPAP.[37]

Although CPAP is typically applied and titrated in a sleep laboratory, autoPAP, which varies positive pressure based on a dynamic algorithm, has come into common use, often as a first-line method of PAP. Because it autotitrates pressure during sleep, it does not require an in-laboratory study with a sleep technician to titrate pressures manually. It also adjusts for variable obstruction related to body position and dynamic changes in airway collapse during sleep.

Surgical and Nonsurgical Options to Facilitate Positive Airway Pressure Use

Although nasal obstruction is usually not the primary source of obstruction in patients with OSA, nasal resistance, increased by septal deviations, hypertrophic inferior turbinates, or internal or external valve collapse, is a predictor of poor CPAP compliance.[38] Nasal obstruction creates more rapid flow and inspiratory pressure leading to increased upper airway collapse, which can make PAP less comfortable because of reduced airflow, rhinitis, dryness, or epistaxis, resulting in poor adherence. Nonsurgical methods such as nasal steroid sprays, Breathe Right strips, nasal dilators, or stents can help improve PAP tolerance. However, when this is inadequate, surgery can be performed to reduce obstruction in the nasal cavity to improve PAP compliance. Inferior turbinate reduction can be performed as an in-office procedure to decrease the size of the turbinates. More definitive reduction can be performed in the operating room, often in combination with a septoplasty to straighten a deviated septum or nasal valve surgery to further open the anterior nose. One study found that average CPAP use increased from 0.5 to 5 hours after septoplasty.[39] In addition, studies have found that nasal surgery to improve nasal airflow is not only effective but also a cost-efficient intervention to improve CPAP adherence and consequent outcomes.[40,41]

Positive Airway Pressure Monitoring and Compliance

The ability to electronically monitor and record nightly use of PAP has revolutionized the treatment of patients with OSA. Previously, adherence was determined by patient report, which was found through covert monitoring to be remarkably unreliable.[42] Without objective monitoring, patients can continue for years with inadequate treatment. With the advent of tracking capabilities on most PAP units, sleep physicians and internists can guide patients toward improved compliance with PAP or escalate to therapies, including oral appliances or surgery. Monitoring has been further incentivized by Medicare and insurance companies, who now refuse to reimburse for PAP units that are not being adequately used.

However, most patients prescribed CPAP are unable to tolerate the mask for the recommended duration, or do not gain adequate benefit from CPAP.[35] Surgical intervention after inadequate response to PAP has been shown to improve quality of life as well as decrease morbidity and mortality.[43] It is incumbent on physicians treating patients with OSA to inform patients of all options for treatment of OSA and decide with the patient what option or what further evaluation may be appropriate.

Oral Appliances

Oral appliances, specifically mandibular repositioning devices, can be used as an initial treatment of patients with mild to moderate OSA and suitable dentition. These devices are typically custom fitted to the upper and lower dentition and advance the lower dentition forward to increase airway diameter and stability. They are comparable with a jaw thrust in moving the tongue forward and tensioning the lateral pharyngeal walls.

The American Academy of Sleep Medicine recommends consideration of oral appliances for patients with OSA who either fail to improve with PAP or are looking for alternative therapies. Meta-analysis has shown no statistically significant difference in the mean reduction in AHI before and after treatment with oral appliances compared with CPAP across all levels of OSA severity; however, for patients with severe OSA, CPAP had greater reduction on AHI compared with oral appliances alone.[44] Mandibular advancement devices can be effective but can exacerbate malocclusion or temporomandibular joint problems. Another type of oral appliance, tongue stabilizing devices, hold the tongue forward by applying suction to the tip of the tongue. These devices can also help with tongue base obstruction; however, they are generally poorly tolerated by patients.[45]

Surgical Intervention in Obstructive Sleep Apnea

Referral for surgical evaluation is appropriate for patients who are inadequately treated by other means or who choose surgical intervention by choice. There are select patients who are excellent candidates for primary surgery, including patients with obstruction from large tonsils or patients with significant retrognathia requiring mandibular advancement. Alternatively, patients with obesity have lower surgical success rates and should be counseled appropriately, possibly including more advanced weight loss strategies or bariatric surgery. Evaluation by a surgical specialist can provide detailed information on treatment options and surgical appropriateness based on the physical examination and apnea severity.

Surgical intervention can be categorized as directly affecting the upper airway patency, muscle tone, or systemic weight. Over the course of the development of sleep surgery, there have been a wide array of surgical techniques to address specific levels of obstruction.

One retrospective study of 20,000 patients found that patients with OSA who used CPAP had higher rates of mortality compared with those who underwent uvulopalatopharyngoplasty (UPPP).[43] Although this includes patients who are both compliant and noncompliant with CPAP, the results powerfully indicate that 1 single surgery for OSA has a measurable effect on mortality. Patients who respond to multilevel surgery have a reduction in inflammation as measured by decreasing C-reactive protein levels, comparable with those who are treated with PAP, providing further evidence of physiologic changes with surgery.[46] These studies support the recommendation by sleep specialists that patients who are unable to tolerate or seek minimal benefit from PAP undergo evaluation for sleep surgery.

SURGERY DIRECTED TO UPPER AIRWAY
Multilevel Surgery

Surgical intervention is commonly required at more than 1 anatomic level. Physical examination, DISE, and patient preference are all integral in the decision making on which surgery to perform. Patients may choose to undergo 1 surgical intervention and reevaluate the severity of sleep disordered breathing, whereas others may choose to undergo multilevel surgery to maximize their success rate during 1 anesthetic. A recent 2020 multicenter randomized controlled trial found that patients with moderate to severe OSA who underwent multilevel surgery to reduce palatal and tongue obstruction had fewer apnea and hypopnea events and decreased patient-reported sleepiness, as measured by the ESS, at 6 months, compared with those who underwent nonsurgical interventions.[47]

NASAL SURGERY
Septoplasty, Polypectomy, Inferior Turbinate Reduction, Rhinoplasty

Surgical intervention to open the nasal passageway has been shown to improve CPAP tolerance and reduce daytime sleepiness as measured by the ESS.[48] Interventions include endoscopic versus open septoplasty to straighten a deviated septum; endoscopic sinus surgery with polypectomy if the patient has comorbid chronic rhinosinusitis with nasal polyposis; turbinate reduction for hypertrophic inferior turbinates; or rhinoplasty to widen the nasal passage and reduce valve collapse. The utility of nasal surgery as a stand-alone procedure to specifically reduce AHI is controversial. A large meta-analysis found that nasal surgery was associated with decreased sleepiness based on the ESS, but no statistically significant decrease in AHI[49]; however, another study found that AHI was reduced when septoplasty was combined with inferior turbinate reduction.[50]

Palate and Velum

Palate and oropharyngeal surgery have undergone significant evolution since the introduction of UPPP in 1981 by Fujita and colleagues.[51] Present surgical intervention includes variations on the original procedure that significantly reduce morbidity and improve outcomes.

Uvulopalatopharyngoplasty

UPPP was once the most commonly performed sleep surgery to address palatal and lateral oropharyngeal collapse, and was found to reduce rates of motor vehicle collisions.[52,53] It is now used selectively and has largely been supplanted by other less morbid and more effective types of pharyngeal surgery.

UPPP involves removing the tonsils, shortening the uvula and soft palate, and resuspending the tonsillar pillars laterally. A landmark literature review found that, for patients with palatal obstruction, 52% had successful outcomes compared with 5% in those with hypopharyngeal obstruction.[54] Consequently, a staging system was developed to predict surgical outcome after UPPP based on anatomy (see **Fig. 1**).[24]

Patients with small tongues and large tonsils had 81% success rates, compared with only 8% for those with large tongues and small tonsils.[24] Studies of this type have underscored the importance of preoperative evaluation of the site of obstruction in order to target surgery appropriately.

Expansion Sphincter Pharyngoplasty

The popularity of UPPP declined because of inconsistent effectiveness, patient morbidity, and prolonged recovery time, whereas the modified expansion sphincter pharyngoplasty (ESP), or functional expansion pharyngoplasty, increased in use. ESP involves a bilateral tonsillectomy with repositioning of pharyngeal muscles to open and stabilize the lateral walls and soft palate. It offers improved success rates compared with UPPP and reduced side effects.[55] A meta-analysis in 2016 showed the overall AHI improved from 40 to 8.3 postoperatively, with an overall success rate of 86.3%.[56]

Tongue Base

Hypopharyngeal obstruction is most commonly caused by an enlarged tongue base, lingual tonsillar hypertrophy, or a collapsed or prolapsing epiglottis. Over the last 15 years, as recognition of retroglossal obstruction has increased, hypopharyngeal surgeries have increased in use.[57] Tongue obstruction is often targeted with tongue radiofrequency to invoke sclerosis and consequent tongue muscle tightening and reduction. Lingual tonsils are often targeted with a lingual tonsillectomy to reduce tongue base obstruction. When the tongue obstruction is caused by prolapse of the tongue posteriorly, genioglossus advancement or genioplasty can be used to pull and tether the muscle of the tongue anteriorly to reduce posterior tongue displacement.

Maxillomandibular Advancement

For patients with midface hypoplasia and retrognathia causing base of tongue obstruction, maxillomandibular advancement is performed. This procedure involves osteotomies of the maxilla and mandible with plate placement to advance the maxilla and mandible anteriorly. The overall surgical success rate is 86.0%, with a 43% OSA cure rate.[58] In patients with isolated oropharyngeal/lateral wall collapse, surgical success was 93%, with AHI decrease from 59.8 to 9.3.[59] The average reduction in AHI ranges between 31 and 51 events per hour, with a mean decrease in AHI of 39.0 events per hour.[60] This surgery comes with significant morbidity and significant postoperative recovery time and is generally reserved for patients who have significant bony disproportion or who have failed other interventions.

Hypoglossal Nerve Stimulator

In recent years, hypoglossal nerve stimulation has become the most popular surgery to target the tongue base, with significant improvement in palatal obstruction as well. This outpatient surgery involves placing an implant pulse generator under the skin of the chest and an electrode in the intercostal space to detect respiration, with a stimulator electrode that implants into the tongue for concomitant tongue protrusion. This surgery is reserved for patients with AHI of 15 to 65, without complete concentric palate collapse on DISE, with at least 75% obstructive apneas. The Stimulation Therapy for Apnea Reduction (STAR) trial evaluating 5-year outcomes found that AHI decreased on average from 33 to 14 with 60% success rate.[61] The Adherence and Outcome of Upper Airway Stimulation for OSA International Registry (ADHERE) database of 508 patients found that AHI decreased from 34 to 7.[62] However, about 15% to 20% of patients cannot tolerate the stimulator despite reprogramming.

Bariatric Surgery

Bariatric surgery, most commonly the Roux-en-Y gastric bypass and sleeve gastrectomy, has been shown to produce significant reduction in BMI, neck circumference, and AHI, compared with standard dietary and exercise regimens.[63] A large meta-analysis of more than 22,000 patients found that more than 80% of those with OSA had improvement or resolution of the OSA postoperatively.[64] Another meta-analysis found that average AHI decreased from 55 to 16, which still warrants additional treatment but is a dramatic improvement.[65]

SUMMARY

OSA is a complex medical disorder with significant impact on mortality, quality of life, and long-term cardiovascular outcomes. OSA is diagnosed on clinical evaluation and a sleep study performed at home or in a sleep laboratory. Although the AHI has been used to quantify severity of disease and treatment success, it does not correlate well with either quality-of-life measures or health outcomes such as hypertension. Therefore, response to treatment should incorporate other metrics as well. OSA can be successfully treated through behavioral, nonsurgical, and surgical methods with improvements in quality of life, morbidity, and mortality. Treatment should be tailored to each individual, and compliance with therapy must be followed to ensure its continued therapeutic value.

Any physician treating patients with OSA should perform a physical examination and make appropriate referrals when questions on anatomic obstruction arise. This assessment may include referral to an otolaryngologist, oral surgeon, dentist who specializes in oral appliances for sleep, or pulmonologist for optimization of treatment of other sleep disorders or PAP management. Surgical intervention should be considered in patients who are noncompliant with or fail PAP use. Improvement in OSA from surgery does not rely on patient compliance and improves mortality and symptoms of OSA even when the PSG does not normalize.

DISCLOSURE

A.N. Goldberg: Keyssa, Inc, consultant and minor stock holder; Siesta Medical, Inc, minor stock holder. Sinus diagnostics and therapeutics, University of California, San Francisco, patent pending 61/624, 105, inventor.

REFERENCES

1. Eckert DJ, Malhotra A. Pathophysiology of adult obstructive sleep apnea. Proc Am Thorac Soc 2008;5(2):144–53.
2. Punjabi NM. The epidemiology of adult obstructive sleep apnea. Proc Am Thorac Soc 2008;5:136–43.
3. Moyer CA, Sonnad SS, Garetz SL, et al. Quality of life in obstructive sleep apnea: a systematic review of the literature. Sleep Med 2001;2:477–91.
4. Redline S, Young T. Epidemiology and natural history of obstructive sleep apnea. Ear Nose Throat J 1993;72(1):20–1, 24-6.
5. Schwab RJ, Gupta KB, Gefter WB, et al. Upper airway and soft tissue anatomy in normal subjects and patients with sleep-disordered breathing. Significance of the lateral pharyngeal walls. Am J Respir Crit Care Med 1995;152(5 Pt 1):1673–89.
6. Strohl KP, Saunders NA, Feldman NT, et al. Obstructive sleep apnea in family members. N Engl J Med 1978;299(18):969–73.

7. Redline S, Tosteson T, Tishler PV, et al. Studies in the genetics of obstructive sleep apnea. Familial aggregation of symptoms associated with sleep-related breathing disturbances. Am Rev Respir Dis 1992;145(2 Pt 1):440–4.

8. Mickelson SA. Nasal surgery for obstructive sleep apnea syndrome. Otolaryngol Clin North Am 2016;49(6):1373–81.

9. Young T, Finn L, Palta M. Chronic nasal congestion at night is a risk factor for snoring in a population-based cohort study. Arch Intern Med 2001;161(12): 1514–9.

10. Greenberg DB. Clinical dimensions of fatigue. Prim Care Companion J Clin Psychiatry 2002;4(3):90–3.

11. Thong JF, Pang KP. Clinical parameters in obstructive sleep apnea: are there any correlations? J Otolaryngol Head Neck Surg 2008;37(6):894–900.

12. Tam S, Woodson BT, Rotenberg B. Outcome measurements in obstructive sleep apnea: beyond the apnea-hypopnea index. Laryngoscope 2014;124(1):337–43.

13. Weaver EM, Kapur V, Yueh B. Polysomnography vs self-reported measures in patients with sleep apnea. Arch Otolaryngol Head Neck Surg 2004;130:453–8.

14. Weaver EM, Woodson BT, Steward DL. Polysomnography indexes are discordant with quality of life, symptoms, and reaction times in sleep apnea patients. Otolaryngol Head Neck Surg 2005;132:255–62.

15. Pang KP, Rotenberg BW. Redefining successful therapy in obstructive sleep apnea: a call to arms. Laryngoscope 2014;124(5):1051–2.

16. Magalang UJ, Dmochowski J, Veeramachaneni S, et al. Prediction of the apnea-hypopnea index from overnight pulse oximetry. Chest 2003;124:1694–701.

17. Nakase-Richardson R, Dahdah MN, Almeida E, et al. Concordance between current American Academy of Sleep Medicine and Centers for Medicare and Medicare scoring criteria for obstructive sleep apnea in hospitalized persons with traumatic brain injury: a VA TBI Model System study. J Clin Sleep Med 2020; 16(6):879–88.

18. Korotinsky A, Assefa SZ, Diaz-Abad M, et al. Comparison of American Academy of Sleep Medicine (AASM) versus Center for Medicare and Medicaid Services (CMS) polysomnography (PSG) scoring rules on AHI and eligibility for continuous positive airway pressure (CPAP) treatment. Sleep Breath 2016;20:1169–74.

19. Peker Y, Hedner J, Kraiczi H, et al. Respiratory disturbance index: an independent predictor of mortality in coronary artery disease. Am J Respir Crit Care Med 2000;162(1):81–6.

20. Johns MW. A new method for measuring daytime sleepiness: the Epworth sleepiness scale. Sleep 1991;14(6):540–5.

21. Kapur VK, Resnick HE, Gottlieb DJ, Sleep Heart Health Study Group. Sleep disordered breathing and hypertension: does self-reported sleepiness modify the association? Sleep 2008;31(8):1127–32.

22. Panoutsopoulos A, Kallianos A, Kostopoulos K, et al. Effect of CPAP treatment on endothelial function and plasma CRP levels in patients with sleep apnea. Med Sci Monit 2012;18(12):CR747–51.

23. Tregear S, Reston J, Schoelles K, et al. Obstructive sleep apnea and risk of motor vehicle crash: systematic review and meta-analysis. J Clin Sleep Med 2009;5(6): 573–81.

24. Friedman M, Ibrahim H, Bass L. Clinical staging for sleep-disordered breathing. Otolaryngol Head Neck Surg 2002;127(1):13–21.

25. Feng Y, Keenan BT, Wang S, et al. Dynamic upper airway imaging during wakefulness in obese subjects with and without sleep apnea. Am J Respir Crit Care Med 2018;198(11):1435–43.

26. Schwab RJ, Pasirstein M, Pierson R, et al. Identification of upper airway anatomic risk factors for obstructive sleep apnea with volumetric magnetic resonance imaging. Am J Respir Crit Care Med 2003;168(5):522–30.
27. Eastwood PR, Platt PR, Shepherd K, et al. Collapsibility of the upper airway at different concentrations of propofol anesthesia. Anesthesiology 2005;103:470–7.
28. Hillman DR, Walsh JH, Maddison KJ, et al. Evolution of changes in upper airway collapsibility during slow induction of anesthesia with propofol. Anesthesiology 2009;111:63–71.
29. Kezirian EJ, Hohenhorst W, de Vries N. Drug-induced sleep endoscopy: the VOTE classification. Eur Arch Otorhinolaryngol 2011;268(8):1233–6.
30. Lee EJ, Cho JH. Meta-analysis of obstruction site observed with drug-induced sleep endoscopy in patients with obstructive sleep apnea. Laryngoscope 2019;129(5):1235–43.
31. Green KK, Kent DT, D'Agostino MA, et al. Drug-induced sleep endoscopy and surgical outcomes: a multicenter cohort study. Laryngoscope 2019;129:761–70.
32. Peppard PE, Young T, Palta M, et al. Longitudinal study of moderate weight change and sleep-disordered breathing. JAMA 2000;284(23):3015–21.
33. Kuna ST, Reboussin DM, Borradaile KE, et al. Long-term effect of weight loss on obstructive sleep apnea severity in obese patients with type 2 diabetes. Sleep 2013;36(5):641–649A.
34. Cowan DC, Livingston E. Obstructive sleep apnoea syndrome and weight loss: review. Sleep Disord 2012;2012:163296.
35. Weaver TE, Grunstein RR. Adherence to continuous positive airway pressure therapy: the challenge to effective treatment. Proc Am Thorac Soc 2008;5:173–8.
36. Peker Y, Glantz H, Eulenburg C, et al. Effect of positive airway pressure on cardiovascular outcomes in coronary artery disease patients with nonsleepy obstructive sleep apnea. The RICCADSA randomized controlled trial. Am J Respir Crit Care Med 2016;194:613–20.
37. George CF. Reduction in motor vehicle collisions following treatment of sleep apnoea with nasal CPAP. Thorax 2001;56(7):508–12.
38. Inoue A, Chiba S, Matsuura K, et al. Nasal function and CPAP compliance. Auris Nasus Larynx 2019;46(4):548–58.
39. Poirier J, George C, Rotenberg B. The effect of nasal surgery on nasal continuous positive airway pressure compliance. Laryngoscope 2014;124(1):317–9.
40. Nakata S, Noda A, Yagi H, et al. Nasal resistance for determinant factor of nasal surgery in CPAP failure patients with obstructive sleep apnea syndrome. Rhinology 2005;43(4):296–9.
41. Kempfle JS, BuSaba NY, Dobrowski JM, et al. A cost-effectiveness analysis of nasal surgery to increase continuous positive airway pressure adherence in sleep apnea patients with nasal obstruction. Laryngoscope 2017;127(4):977–83.
42. Kribbs NB, Pack AI, Kline LR, et al. Objective measurement of patterns of nasal CPAP use by patients with obstructive sleep apnea. Am Rev Respir Dis 1993;147(4):887–95.
43. Weaver EM, Maynard C, Yueh B. Survival of veterans with sleep apnea: continuous positive airway pressure versus surgery. Otolaryngol Head Neck Surg 2004;130(6):659–65.
44. Ramar K, Dort LC, Katz SG, et al. Clinical practice guideline for the treatment of obstructive sleep apnea and snoring with oral appliance therapy: an update for 2015. J Clin Sleep Med 2015;11(7):773–827.
45. Deane SA, Cistulli PA, Ng AT, et al. Comparison of mandibular advancement splint and tongue stabilizing device in obstructive sleep apnea: a randomized

controlled trial [published correction appears in Sleep. 2009 Aug 1;32(8):table of contents]. Sleep 2009;32(5):648–53.

46. Kezirian EJ, Malhotra A, Goldberg AN, et al. Changes in obstructive sleep apnea severity, biomarkers, and quality of life after multilevel surgery. Laryngoscope 2010;120(7):1481–8.

47. MacKay S, Carney AS, Catcheside PG, et al. Effect of multilevel upper airway surgery vs medical management on the apnea-hypopnea index and patient-reported daytime sleepiness among patients with moderate or severe obstructive sleep apnea: The SAMS randomized clinical trial. JAMA 2020;324(12):1168–79.

48. Li HY, Lee LA, Wang PC, et al. Can nasal surgery improve obstructive sleep apnea: subjective or objective? Am J Rhinol Allergy 2009;23:e51–5.

49. Li H-Y, Wang P-C, Chen Y-P, et al. Critical appraisal and meta-analysis of nasal surgery for obstructive sleep apnea. Am J Rhinol Allergy 2011;25(1):45–9.

50. Moxness MH, Nordgård S. An observational cohort study of the effects of septoplasty with or without inferior turbinate reduction in patients with obstructive sleep apnea. BMC Ear Nose Throat Disord 2014;14:11.

51. Fujita S, Conway W, Zorick F, et al. Surgical correction of anatomic abnormalities in obstructive sleep apnea syndrome: uvulopalatopharyngoplasty. Otolaryngol Head Neck Surg 1981;89(6):923–34.

52. Haraldsson PO, Carenfelt C, Lysdahl M, et al. Long-term effect of uvulopalatopharyngoplasty on driving performance. Arch Otolaryngol Head Neck Surg 1995;121(1):90–4.

53. Haraldsson PO, Carenfelt C, Lysdahl M, et al. Does uvulopalatopharyngoplasty inhibit automobile accidents? Laryngoscope 1995;105(6):657–61.

54. Sher AE, Thorpy MJ, Shprintzen RJ, et al. Predictive value of Muller maneuver in selection of patients for uvulopalatopharyngoplasty. Laryngoscope 1985;95:1483–7.

55. Pang KP, Woodson BT. Expansion sphincter pharyngoplasty: a new technique for the treatment of obstructive sleep apnea. Otolaryngol Head Neck Surg 2007;137(1):110–4.

56. Pang KP, Pang EB, Win MT, et al. Expansion sphincter pharyngoplasty for the treatment of OSA: a systemic review and meta-analysis. Eur Arch Otorhinolaryngol 2016;273(9):2329–33.

57. Kezirian EJ, Maselli J, Vittinghoff E, et al. Obstructive sleep apnea surgery practice patterns in the United States: 2000 to 2006. Otolaryngol Head Neck Surg 2010;143(3):441–7.

58. Holty JE, Guilleminault C. Maxillomandibular advancement for the treatment of obstructive sleep apnea: a systematic review and meta-analysis. Sleep Med Rev 2010;14(5):287–97.

59. Liu SY, Huon LK, Powell NB, et al. Lateral pharyngeal wall tension after maxillomandibular advancement for obstructive sleep apnea is a marker for surgical success: observations from drug-induced sleep endoscopy. J Oral Maxillofac Surg 2015;73(8):1575–82.

60. Giralt-Hernando M, Valls-Ontañón A, Guijarro-Martínez R, et al. Impact of surgical maxillomandibular advancement upon pharyngeal airway volume and the apnoea-hypopnoea index in the treatment of obstructive sleep apnoea: systematic review and meta-analysis. BMJ Open Respir Res 2019;6(1):e000402.

61. Woodson BT, Strohl KP, Soose RJ, et al. Upper airway stimulation for obstructive sleep apnea: 5-year outcomes. Otolaryngol Head Neck Surg 2018;159(1):194–202.

62. Heiser C, Steffen A, Boon M, et al. Post-approval upper airway stimulation predictors of treatment effectiveness in the ADHERE registry. Eur Respir J 2019;53(1): 1801405.

63. Ashrafian H, Toma T, Rowland SP, et al. Bariatric surgery or non-surgical weight loss for obstructive sleep apnoea? a systematic review and comparison of meta-analyses. Obes Surg 2015;25(7):1239–50.

64. Buchwald H, Avidor Y, Braunwald E, et al. Bariatric surgery: a systematic review and meta-analysis. JAMA 2004;292(14):1724–37. Erratum in: JAMA. 2005 Apr 13;293(14):1728.

65. Greenburg DL, Lettieri CJ, Eliasson AH. Effects of surgical weight loss on measures of obstructive sleep apnea: a meta-analysis. Am J Med 2009;122(6): 535–42.

Vertigo

Streamlining the Evaluation through Symptom Localization

Kimberley S. Noij, MD, PhD[a,b], Scott B. Shapiro, MD[c],
Ravi N. Samy, MD[c], James G. Naples, MD[a,b],*

KEYWORDS

- Vertigo • Peripheral vestibular disorders • Central vestibular disorders
- Vestibular examination

KEY POINTS

- Vertigo is the illusion of internal or external motion. It is not a diagnosis, and the symptom alone, independent of other historical factors, offers little insight into the source of the problem.
- Differentiating the organ system responsible for dizziness symptoms is a helpful first step in the evaluation of patients with this complaint. Localizing the problem is often more important than providing a specific diagnosis.
- True vertigo often has its origins in the central nervous system or peripheral nervous system; identification of the location of origin can streamline the workup.
- Imaging and vestibular testing should be used as an adjunct to a comprehensive history to assist in localization and to rule out disorders.
- Regardless of the source of symptoms, the mainstay of treatment for vertigo-induced pathology is physical therapy.

 Video content accompanies this article at http://www.medical.theclinics.com.

INTRODUCTION
Definitions

Before the discussion of evaluation and work up for the vertiginous patient, this article clarifies what is meant by the symptom of vertigo. The strict definition of vertigo is the illusion of internal motion when no motion is occurring.[1] The number of descriptions

[a] Department of Surgery, Beth Israel Deaconess Medical Center, Boston, MA, USA;
[b] Department of Otolaryngology Head and Neck Surgery, Beth Israel Deaconess Medical Center, Harvard Medical School, Boston, MA, USA; [c] Department of Otolaryngology–Head and Neck Surgery, University of Cincinnati College of Medicine, Cincinnati, OH, USA
* Corresponding author. Department of Otolaryngology-Head and Neck Surgery, Beth Israel Deaconess Medical Center, Harvard Medical School, 85 Binney St, Boston, MA 02215.
E-mail address: jnaples@bidmc.harvard.edu

Med Clin N Am 105 (2021) 901–916
https://doi.org/10.1016/j.mcna.2021.05.011
0025-7125/21/© 2021 Elsevier Inc. All rights reserved.

medical.theclinics.com

patients provide for this symptom are too diverse to list here, but often people will describe the sensation of room spinning or describe their world moving despite the fact that they remain stationary. The word dizziness is often used as a descriptor, but this does not define vertigo. Similarly, light-headedness and imbalance may be descriptive terms that offer little insight to the problem. It is incumbent upon the physician to understand the context of symptoms within the framework of the patient's history to offer the appropriate workup.

Many of the references we provide offer information regarding dizziness. Research on disorders causing vertigo is often disease-specific and provides details beyond the scope of this article. As such, the word dizziness may be used more broadly to encompass vertiginous patients; however, it is important recognize that not all dizziness is vertigo.

Background

This article describes the evaluation of patients with vertigo and provides the primary care physician (PCP) a framework for diagnostic considerations. Yearly, an estimated 33.4 million adults (14.8%) in the United States suffer from dizziness.[2] Dizziness accounts for about 5% of primary care visits and about 4% of emergency department visits.[3,4] The yearly national cost for patients presenting with dizziness in US emergency rooms have been estimated to exceed $4 billion.[4] Dizziness is a generic symptom that typically includes blurring of vision, lightheadedness, unsteadiness, floating sensation, tilting sensation, and vertigo.[1] Within the chief complaint of dizziness, vertigo accounts for between 25% and 54% of cases.[5,6] The evaluation of dizzy patients is challenging owing to the breadth of descriptions patients provide for their symptoms and the complexity of the pathways responsible for maintaining balance. In general, balance is maintained by integrating vision, proprioception, and vestibular (inner ear) function in the central nervous system (**Fig. 1**). A problem with any of these systems can cause dizziness. Therefore, the choice of diagnostics and treatment can vary widely between patients. Determining which systems are involved and localizing the problem is the most important part of the evaluation of these patients because this

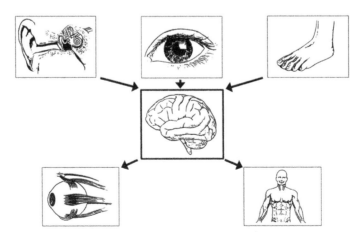

Fig. 1. There are various sensory inputs that contribute to our sense of balance that include the peripheral vestibular system, inner ear, visual system, musculoskeletal system, and proprioceptive input. These systems and sensory inputs are integrated in the central nervous system, and deficits in any of these systems can lead to the perception of dizziness.

will (1) aid in decision making regarding further testing, (2) determine whether imaging is necessary, (3) help to clarify when patient referral is indicated, and (4) determine which specialist to refer to.

This article highlights that, for the PCP, providing a specific diagnosis for the dizzy patient is not as important as symptom localization. Dizziness is a nonspecific symptom and, as such, early attempts to provide a specific diagnosis may lead the PCP to overlook other possible etiologies. Instead, symptom localization maintains a less specific approach that can guide further workup. Symptom localization is most efficiently accomplished by taking a comprehensive history that focuses on specific questions related to each of the potential organ systems involved in balance. In this article, an algorithm for symptom localization and a streamlined approach for the workup of vertigo are provided. Finally, the most common central and peripheral vestibular disorders seen in the outpatient setting are discussed.

TAKING A MEDICAL HISTORY IN THE DIZZY PATIENT: A SYSTEMS-BASED APPROACH

There are various proposed algorithms to assist the physician in history taking of the dizzy patient. Traditionally, the focus has been on clarifying what the patient means by their symptoms, the timing of their symptoms, duration of their symptoms, and so on. More recent work suggests that the characterization of dizziness is less relevant than the timing and potential triggers.[6] In conjunction with a history that roughly defines the duration of symptoms and potential triggers, a systems-based approach to further history taking will lead to an efficient workup. This article focusses on the evaluation of dizziness as the chief complaint. Although there are innumerable systemic and focal disorders that present with dizziness as an associated symptom, it is beyond the scope of this article to review every possible cause of dizziness.

Otologic-Specific History

Many of the peripheral (otologic) causes of dizziness are accompanied by otologic-specific symptoms. In addition to the onset, duration, intensity, frequency, and progression of vertigo, it is important to inquire about precipitating factors, previous episodes, and associated symptoms. Associated symptoms that should specifically be asked for include hearing loss, tinnitus, autophony (unusually loud or disturbing sound of one's own voice),[7] and hyperacusis (marked intolerance to ordinary environmental sounds).[8] Patients with associated auditory symptoms are more likely to have a peripheral problem.[9] More so, unilateral otologic symptoms would be even more convincing for a likely peripheral otologic source because bilateral tinnitus and hearing loss can be seen in a large percentage of the population without identifiable pathology. For example, in considering a patient with possible Meniere disease, the combination of episodic vertigo lasting for hours, hearing loss, and tinnitus or aural fullness should direct the PCP to pursue audiometric and otolaryngologic evaluation, irrespective of the type of vertigo described. This example highlights the importance of asking the patient about hearing loss and tinnitus as it results in appropriate evaluation, which eventually will result in a correct diagnosis.

Central Nervous System–Specific History

It is uncommon for acute, neurologic sources of vertigo to present to the PCP. Instead, these patients often present to the emergency room.[6] More often, the outpatient presentation of central vertigo is chronic, episodic, or recurrent. Symptoms of patients with central sources of vertigo are often complex and confusing. As such, the main priority for the PCP should be to rule out stroke or transient ischemic attack, and the

ABCD2 score (calculated based on age, blood pressure, clinical features, duration of symptoms, and history of diabetes) is a facile way to determine the associated risk for stroke.[10] Focal neurologic symptoms associated with the vertigo should also raise concern for a central cause. Finally, visual changes or bowel or bladder changes should be discussed because they can be present in demyelinating disorders. Vertigo or dizziness as a symptom of stroke traditionally occurs without specific triggers and is nonpositional. However, other central processes in the posterior fossa can present with dizziness triggered by changes in position.[10,11]

Besides stroke, other central sources should be explored. Headache symptoms are relevant because, in combination with vertigo or dizziness, this symptom could point to a number of disorders (eg, idiopathic intracranial hypertension, Chiari malformation, and migraine).[11–13] Patients may describe a history of migraine or a family history of migraine, and symptoms do not always accompany vertigo specifically. Although some patients with migraine identify symptom triggers, many do not. Additionally, a history of light or sound sensitivity can increase suspicion for vestibular migraine.[13]

The central nervous system history is often the most complicated and confusing. The range of possible causes is immense, and the diagnoses range from life threatening to benign. As stated elsewhere in this article, arriving at a specific diagnosis is not as important as being suspicious for a central source because localizing the pathology leads to an appropriate workup.

Other Organ System-Based Histories (Cardiac, Musculoskeletal, Psychiatric) and Medications

Commonly, patients present with symptoms of vertigo or dizziness that are due to sources other than the peripheral or central vestibular systems. The cardiac, musculoskeletal, and psychiatric histories are important to evaluate when a peripheral otologic or central source seems unlikely. Patients with labile blood pressure commonly have symptoms of dizziness, which may be triggered by standing from a seated position. Similarly, patients with cardiac arrhythmias may have symptoms that precipitate an evaluation by the PCP. Patients with peripheral neuropathy and other mobility concerns will often describe symptoms of imbalance and dizziness. Recall that proprioception is one of the key inputs that are integrated to help maintain balance. As such, it is common for patients with diabetes and spinal column issues to describe dizziness.

Beyond the cardiac and musculoskeletal systems, vertigo and dizziness are commonly associated with psychiatric disorders such as anxiety and depression.[14] It is important to determine the role of these coexisting conditions because control of these symptoms may benefit the patient. Although treating comorbid conditions is often necessary, caution needs to be exercised when medicating patients, because many medications have side effects that include dizziness, which may exacerbate the patient's condition. Polypharmacy is likely an under-recognized source of dizziness, and judicious management of this is important to overall care of the dizzy patient.[15]

PHYSICAL EXAMINATION

Patients with vertigo often have few, if any, abnormal physical examination findings. However, there are subtle examination findings that can aid the physician in localization of the symptom and point toward a central or peripheral source of vertigo.

In addition to a comprehensive past medical, surgical, social, and family history, there are specific systems that require additional attention in evaluation of the dizzy patient.

- Cardiovascular examination
- Otologic examination
- Neurologic examination
- Review of medications and psychiatric comorbidities
- Focused vestibular examination

We review details of the focused vestibular examination, because this is the highest yield in localizing the source of the problem. The history largely dictates which other components of the examination should be performed (**Table 1**).

Focused Vestibular Examination

The most relevant part of the physical examination involves specific maneuvers that evaluate the vestibular system. The simplest evaluation is observation of the eyes looking for nystagmus. If nystagmus is present, it offers significant insights to whether the problem is one of peripheral or central origin. Nystagmus has a slow- and fast-phase component, and the direction of the fast phase is used to describe the nystagmus. Peripheral nystagmus is different from central nystagmus in 3 essential ways. Peripheral nystagmus:

1. Is latent in onset,
2. Fatigues, and
3. Can be suppressed with visual fixation.

These clues can help the examiner to localize the problem. In addition, vertical or down-beating nystagmus is almost always representative of a central disorder (eg, Arnold-Chiari malformation), whereas spontaneous horizontal nystagmus can represent a peripheral problem that follows an acute peripheral insult (eg, labyrinthitis) (**Fig. 2** and Video 1).[11,16] It is important to note that gaze evoked nystagmus, also referred to as end point nystagmus, can be found in healthy individuals and occurs with ocular displacement greater than 30° from center.

The Head Impulse Test (HIT) evaluates the vestibulo-ocular reflex. This valuable test evaluates eye movement and provides information regarding the integrity of the peripheral vestibular system. During the HIT, the patient focuses on a target in front of them (such as the examiner's nose). The examiner quickly rotates the head to the left or right, while the patient should attempt to remain focused on the target, and observes eye movement. The test is considered abnormal if the patient is unable

---

Table 1
Key components of the physical examination of the dizzy patient

Physical Examination	Components
1. Focused vestibular examination	HINTS (Head Impulse Test, nystagmus and test of skew), Dix-Hallpike
2. Otologic examination	Otoscopy, Rinne, Weber
3. Neurologic examination	Mental status, cranial nerves, cerebellar examination, sensation, motor system, coordination, station/gait
4. Cardiovascular examination	Orthostatic blood pressure evaluation, tilt table test, auscultation of carotid arteries
5. Other	Review medication list and polypharmacy, co-morbid psychiatric disorders (anxiety, depression, panic attacks)

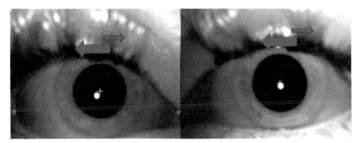

Fig. 2. Spontaneous right-beating horizontal nystagmus. After an acute left insult such as labyrinthitis, patients may have findings of spontaneous horizontal nystagmus toward the unaffected ear. The large arrow represents the fast-phase, right-beating horizontal nystagmus. The small arrow represents the slow-phase of the nystagmus. See Video 1.

maintain focus on the target and requires a corrective eye movement (**Fig. 3**). Patients with a unilateral vestibular loss make a corrective eye movement when the head is rotated toward the side of the lesion. Patients with central lesions will show a normal HIT result. When the HIT is combined with evaluation of skew deviation, it can be both sensitive and specific in determining whether the lesion is located in the peripheral or central vestibular system. During this test, one of the patient's eyes is covered for several seconds and then quickly uncovered. If the previously covered eye makes a corrective movement in the vertical plane, this movement indicates a central issue, such as a cerebellar stroke. This test is then repeated for the other eye. Despite the

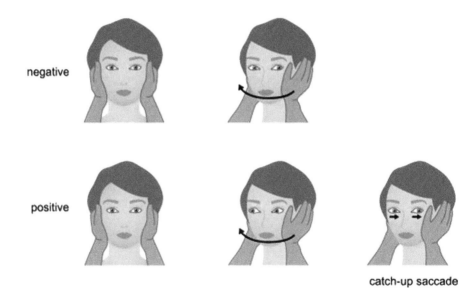

catch-up saccade

Fig. 3. Head Impulse Test (HIT). A HIT can be used to identify a peripheral vestibular insult. The examiner should turn the head quickly to the left and right, and ask the patient to focus their vision on a target such as the examiner's nose. When turning the head to the normal side (*top*), the eyes fixate on the target. When turning to the affected side (*bottom*), the eyes do not fixate on the target, and make a corrective saccade back toward the target. (With permission D. Straumann. Bedside Examination. Handbook of Clinical Neurology. 2016; Vol 137, Figure 7.3.)

high sensitivity and specificity with the addition of skew testing, identification of skew can be challenging without experience. Therefore, the interpretation of this examination can be challenging.[17]

The last test of the focused vestibular examination is the Dix–Hallpike maneuver. This maneuver is used as a diagnostic tool in the evaluation of benign paroxysmal positional vertigo (BPPV). It should be performed at the end of the examination, because a positive Dix–Hallpike test causes dizziness and may limit a patient's ability to participate with the rest of the evaluation. During the Dix–Hallpike test, the patient is seated on an examination table. The examiner holds the patient's head with both hands and turns it 45° from the midline. Then with eyes open, the examiner rapidly directs the patient into a supine position with the head extending over the edge of the examination table. Instruct the patient to keep eyes open and observe for nystagmus for approximately 45 to 60 seconds. The occurrence of vertigo and/or nystagmus indicates a positive test. The direction of the nystagmus can provide information as to the location of the problem, although this factor may be difficult to appreciate. A rotatory and upbeat nystagmus the affected ear down that is latent in onset and fatigable indicates BPPV of the posterior semicircular canal (**Fig. 4**, Video 2).[18,19] Although other forms of nystagmus can be seen with the involvement of the other canals during this maneuver, BPPV of the posterior canal is the most common type.[19] If the Dix–Hallpike test suggests BPPV of the posterior semicircular canal, a therapeutic Epley maneuver can be performed in the office (**Fig. 5**).[20] A lack of symptom improvement with repeated Epley maneuvers requires reevaluation and should raise suspicion of BPPV within another canal or another possible pathology. BPPV seems to be associated with osteoporosis and osteopenia.[21]

WORKUP AND SOURCE OF SYMPTOMS

Once the history and physical examination are completed, decisions regarding the workup and management should be dictated by abnormal findings of a specific organ system and not by a specific potential diagnosis (**Figs. 6 and 7**). Although clinicians often prioritize specific diagnoses on their differential, it is necessary to keep other diagnostic considerations in mind. The remainder of this article focusses on the workup for peripheral and central sources of dizziness. Because it may not always be obvious which organ system(s) is/are involved, evaluation by multiple specialists to rule out the contribution of a specific organ system may be necessary. This requires patience from both the patient and the referring physician or PCP.

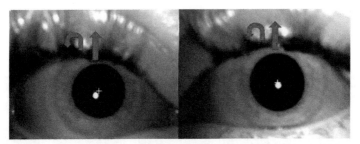

Fig. 4. Right posterior canal BPPV. In BPPV of the posterior semicircular canal, the characteristic nystagmus is up-beating and rotatory (*arrows*) when the affected ear is placed downward in the Dix–Hallpike position. Note that other variations of eye movements are possible, and BPPV of the posterior canal is the most common variant. See Video 2.

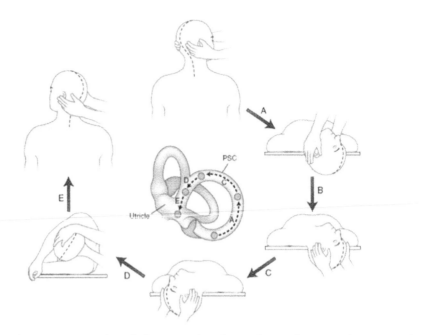

Fig. 5. Epley maneuver. A Dix–Hallpike suggestive of posterior canal BPPV can be converted to the therapeutic Epley maneuver. The maneuver aims to reposition the displaced otoconia to the macula of the utricle. (With permission Kirber KA. Vertigo and Dizziness in the Emergency Department. Emerg Med Clin North Am. 2009 February ; 27(1). Figure 2).

Peripheral and Otologic Workup and Differential Diagnosis

Patients suspected of having a otologic or peripheral vestibular pathology will likely require evaluation by an otolaryngologist. Unless symptoms are consistent with BPPV (discussed elsewhere in this article), most of the peripheral (otologic) sources of vertigo necessitate audiometric evaluation. Often patients are not completely aware of the degree of hearing loss, and they may have difficulty identifying their hearing loss in the acute phase of vertigo. Nonetheless, in many peripheral otologic disorders hearing loss is a key symptom for diagnosis (eg, Meniere disease, labyrinthitis) (**Table 2**).

Additionally, comprehensive vestibular testing and imaging may also be performed as necessary. The goal of vestibular testing is to objectify the function of the vestibular

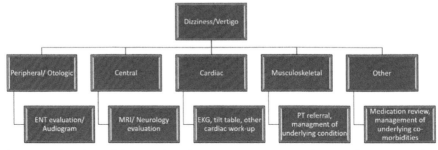

Fig. 6. Initial workup of dizziness based on organ-system. EKG, electrocardiogram; PT, physical therapy.

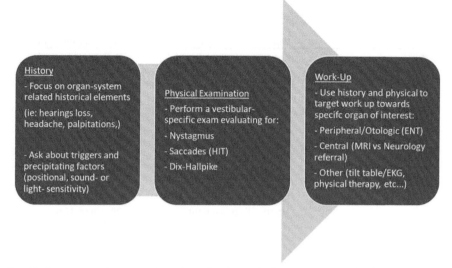

History
- Focus on organ-system related historical elements
(ie: hearings loss, headache, palpitations,)

- Ask about triggers and precipitating factors (positional, sound- or light- sensitivity)

Physical Examination
- Perform a vestibular-specific exam evaluating for:
- Nystagmus
- Saccades (HIT)
- Dix-Hallpike

Work-Up
- Use history and physical to target work up towards specifc organ of interest:
- Peripheral/Otologic (ENT)
- Central (MRI vs Neurology referral)
- Other (tilt table/EKG, physical therapy, etc...)

Fig. 7. Summary of systems-based evaluation of the patients with dizziness. EKG, electrocardiogram.

system and attempt to localize and differentiate central from peripheral sources. A detailed description of vestibular testing is beyond the scope of this article. **Table 2** outlines the most common peripheral/otologic sources of dizziness and suggested workup.

Central Workup

If the history and physical examination raise suspicion for the presence of central pathology, a computed tomography scan and/or MRI is likely warranted. If there is concern for an acute insult, evaluation in an emergency room setting is required. A challenge in the evaluation of central sources of dizziness is that imaging findings may not always be present, and the history may provide the clue to a specific diagnosis. Evaluation by a neurologist or other specialist may be necessary to workup specific causes of central vertigo/dizziness, especially if imaging does not reveal specific pathology. **Table 3** outlines some of the central sources of dizziness and suggested workup considerations. This list is certainly not comprehensive, but it does highlight some of the key historical features that point toward a central source.

Other

The list of other sources of dizziness is long, and what is presented here is not intended to be exhaustive. Instead, the most common sources of nonperipheral and noncentral dizziness are highlighted. Systemic disorders that may produce dizziness such as acute medication toxicities, hyperglycemia or hypoglycemia, and various infectious disorders are not necessarily included here because their presentation is variable and dizziness is rarely the chief complaint.

If a cardiac origin of dizziness is suspected, several additional tests are indicated, such as orthostatic blood pressure measurement (eg, a tilt table test), and electrocardiogram, echocardiogram, and evaluation by a cardiologist. Patients with dizziness of musculoskeletal origin benefit from physical therapy. If underlying anxiety or depression seems to play a role, initiation of antidepressants may be beneficial.[14,15,22,23]

Table 2
Common peripheral vestibular disorders

	Clinical Presentation	Workup and Examination
BPPV[19]	Room-spinning vertigo Seconds in duration Precipitated by position (often lying down or turning in bed)	Dix–Hallpike: diagnostic tool Epley maneuver: therapeutic (for posterior canal BPPV)
Meniere's disease[37]	*Episodic* vertigo lasting for hours Associated with **unilateral hearing loss** and **aural fullness** **Unilateral tinnitus** Symptoms *fluctuate* No specific precipitant	Otolaryngology consult Audiometry With or without vestibular testing MRI Clinical criteria[37]: Two episodes of vertigo 20 min to 12 h Audiometrically documented SHNL[a] Fluctuating tinnitus, aural fullness or hearing loss
Vestibular neuritis/ labyrinthitis[38,39]	Room spinning vertigo lasting for ≥24 h With or without **unilateral hearing loss** and **tinnitus** Labyrinthitis includes **hearing LOSS** and/or **tinnitus** Neuritis does not include hearing loss or tinnitus Often without identified precipitant	Often requires emergency-level care for hydration and emesis control Consider otolaryngology consult in postacute phase Audiometry With or without vestibular testing With or without MRI Spontaneous nystagmus (acute phase): fast-beat nystagmus directed toward unaffected ear HINTS examination (postacute phase): HIT with catch up saccade No skew deviation
Superior semicircular canal dehiscence syndrome[40]	**Sound-** or **pressure-**induced dizziness **Autophony** **Pulsatile tinnitus** **Hyperacusis** Bizarre symptoms such as "hearing eye movement"	Otolaryngology consult Audiometry Vestibular testing (VEMP) Computed tomography scan of the temporal bones (oriented in planes parallel and perpendicular to superior semicircular canal)

(continued on next page)

Table 2
(continued)

	Clinical Presentation	Workup and Examination
Vestibular schwannoma[41]	Gradual onset of **hearing loss, tinnitus** and imbalance	Otolaryngology consult Audiometry: asymmetric SNHL and/or speech perception score ABR: increased latency MRI of the internal auditory canal

Abbreviations: ABR: auditory brainstem response; BPPV, benign paroxysmal positional vertigo; HINTS, Head Impulse Test, nystagmus and test of skew; HIT, Head Impulse Test; SNHL, sensorineural hearing loss; VEMP, vestibular evoked myogenic potential.

Note that this list is not comprehensive, rather it outlines the most common peripheral vestibular disorders. Organ-system specific symptoms are presented in **Bold** font to highlight that many peripheral otologic disorders are associated with complaints related to hearing, tinnitus, or aural fullness.

[a] Sensorineural hearing loss audiometrically documented and defined as a bone-conduction threshold $\geq$30 dB HL at 2 consecutive frequencies of <2000 Hz.

- *Cardiac Sources:* Hypotension or arrhythmia[24,25]
  - Often associated with standing from seated position
  - Precipitated by sitting up (not lying down)
  - Patients often describe cardiac history with blood pressure control issues, start of new hypertension medication, or a history of arrhythmias
  - Orthostatic blood pressures or electrocardiogram needed
  - Therapy aimed at underlying source
- Peripheral postural perceptual dizziness[26,27]
  - Chronic imbalance (>3 months)
  - Often starts after acute dizziness attack
  - Exacerbated by visual stimuli and visually rich environments (driving on highway, grocery store)
  - Often seen with comorbid anxiety and/or depression
  - Physical therapy and antidepressants are treatment options
- Cervicogenic dizziness[28]
  - Chronic dizziness
  - Often associated with headache and neck pain
  - Cervical spine issues common
  - Headache is tension type and thus different from migraine
- Anxiety or panic attack[29]
  - History of anxiety is important
  - Usually precipitated by specific situational trigger
  - Often coexists with another dizziness-related disorder
  - Treatment and control of this comorbidity may alleviate dizziness symptoms
- Mal de débarquement syndrome [30]
  - Need to solidify history of cruise or boat trip
  - Chronic imbalance or "swaying sensation"
  - Worse when still or lying down
  - Treatment consists of physical therapy
- Musculoskeletal source or peripheral neuropathy[22,31]

Table 3
Central vestibular disorders

	Clinical Presentation	Workup and Examination
Transient ischemic attack/ vascular insult[17]	Vertigo of variable duration: Lasting minutes to days. Unprecipitated by position. **Variable neurologic symptoms based on the location of the insult**: Ataxia. **Headache**. Speech-finding difficulties	If concern for vascular insult, immediate work up in an emergency setting is warranted. Computed tomography scan of the head. MRI of the head. Stroke team consult. **HINTS** examination. Skew deviation. Normal Head Impulse Test. Direction-changing nystagmus
Vestibular migraine[35,42]	Episodic dizziness or room-spinning vertigo lasting hours to days. History of migraine. **Headache** and migraine features >50% of episodes. Photophobia and/or phonophobia. Other triggers, such as Wine, Caffeine, Insomnia	ICDH-3 criteria. Need to rule out other sources such as vascular insult. With or without MRI. Medical management, such as beta-blockers, SNRIs, antiepileptics
Chiari Malformation[11]	Episodic or chronic dizziness. **Headache**. Precipitated by increases in intracranial pressure: Lying down, Cough/Sneeze, Straining	Persistent down-beating nystagmus. Can be worse when supine (eg, Dix-Hallpike maneuver). MRI necessary for diagnosis. Neurosurgery consult
Demyelinating disorder[43,44]	Episodic vertigo. **Accompanied by other neurologic symptoms**: Incontinence, Visual deficits, Impaired coordination, Other	MS: McDonald criteria. MRI. Neurology consult
IIH[12]	Chronic dizziness and ataxia. **Various other neurologic Symptoms**: Headache, Visual disturbance, Neck stiffness, Nausea	MRI. Lumbar puncture to measure opening pressure, which is high in IIH. Neuro-ophthalmologic evaluation

Abbreviations: HINTS, Head Impulse Test, nystagmus and test of skew; ICDH, International Classification of Headache Disorders; IIH, idiopathic intracranial hypertension; MS, multiple sclerosis; SNRI, serotonin–norepinephrine reuptake inhibitor.

Note that this list is not comprehensive, rather it outlines the more common central vestibular disorders. Organ-system specific symptoms are presented in **Bold** font to highlight that many central vestibular disorders are associated with complaints related to the central nervous system.

- o Recall that proprioception is an essential component of the sensory input that contributes to balance; as such, patients with musculoskeletal problems pr neuropathy often present with imbalance or dizziness
- o Patients are often elderly or obese (chronic osteoarthritis, osteoporosis)
- o Suspect in diabetic patient and patients with a history of back pain or spinal cord issues
- o Treatment of underlying source is essential
- o Physical therapy is helpful in the presence of a spinal source
- Polypharmacy or ototoxicity[15,32,33]
  - o Examples of ototoxic medications are aminoglycoside antibiotics (tobramycin, gentamicin), loop diuretics, and certain chemotherapeutic agents (cisplatin, carboplatin, vincristine); interestingly, almost all medications list dizziness as a side effect
  - o Meclizine is commonly used to control symptoms of acute dizziness and vertigo; it is an antihistamine that has a sedative effect and can thus exacerbate symptoms, especially in the elderly population
  - o Polypharmacy is likely under-recognized. Multidrug class medication list or multiple drugs of the same class can contribute
  - o Remove or adjust offending agent

TREATMENT

Therapies for the various disorders are often targeted at the underlying cause, many of which are beyond the scope of the PCP. Diagnosis of a specific cause and targeted therapy should not necessarily be the goal of evaluation in the primary care setting. A therapy that is, beneficial for the majority of patients presenting with dizziness/vertigo is physical therapy. The physical therapist can address coping strategies and prevent falls in a wide-range of dizziness-related disorders, including peripheral vestibulopathies, BPPV, migraine, stoke rehabilitation, musculoskeletal disorders, neuropathies, and so on.[23] It is helpful for the physical therapist to provide a suspected source of dizziness because this information allows them to tailor their therapy. For example, vestibular therapy for patients suffering from peripheral vestibular pathology is very different from therapy for patients with proprioceptive issues. Physical therapists can be more efficient in their treatment planning with some background information from the referring physician before the patient's visit.

From the PCP's perspective, patients with dizziness who do not require emergent evaluation or acute central vascular workup, physical therapy can be initiated while referral to a specialist is pending. This practice can facilitate recovery and improve the patient's functional abilities while awaiting specific diagnostic tests or evaluation.

In addition to physical therapy, an important therapeutic consideration for dizziness is medical management. As discussed elsewhere in this article, meclizine is commonly prescribed for acute dizziness-related disorders, and can contribute to the problem owing to its sedative side-effects.[34] Selective serotonin reuptake inhibitors or serotonin–norepinephrine reuptake inhibitors have been used with variable rates of success in disorders such as migraine, peripheral postural perceptual dizziness, and may help to control comorbid anxiety and depressive symptoms that often accompany dizziness-related disorders.[35,36]

Finally, it is important to realize when patient referral for additional testing and management is appropriate. The complexities of the vestibular system are hard to overstate and patients may require evaluations with multiple specialists as no one specialty "owns" dizziness. Despite this circumstance, an organ systems–based approach to the history and a vestibular-specific examination can streamline the evaluation of patients with dizziness. Counseling patients on the potential necessity for multiple evaluations and tests can set appropriate expectations as they navigate the complex workup.

SUMMARY

The workup of dizziness can be complicated, because multiple organ systems are involved with balance. In the primary care setting, symptom localization is more important than reaching a specific diagnosis. Localization of the problem starts with a thorough history focusing on organ-specific associated symptoms and a vestibular-specific examination. These simple approaches will help the PCP to differentiate peripheral from central and other sources of dizziness. Once a suspected location of the problem is identified, workup and management can be targeted to a specific organ system (Dix–Hallpike, audiogram, MRI, physical therapy, etc) and referrals to the appropriate specialists made (otolaryngology, neurology, cardiology, etc). This article provides a streamlined approach to evaluating the dizzy patient and aimed to improve efficiency.

CLINICS CARE POINTS

- The main goal in evaluating a patient with dizziness/vertigo is localization of symptoms (ie, peripheral vs central vs other).
- A targeted, vestibular-specific examination can assist in localizing the lesion.
- Symptom localization can streamline the workup by facilitating appropriate referrals and initiation of therapy.

DISCLOSURE

No conflict of interest to disclose (K.S. Noij, S.B. Shapiro, J.G. Naples). Research funding from Cochlear Americas (R.N. Samy).

SUPPLEMENTARY DATA

Supplementary data to this article can be found online at https://doi.org/10.1016/j.mcna.2021.05.011.

REFERENCES

1. Bisdorff A, Von Brevern M, Lempert T, et al. Classification of vestibular symptoms: towards an international classification of vestibular disorders. J Vestib Res 2009; 19:1–13.
2. Kerber KA, Callaghan BC, Telian SA, et al. Dizziness symptom type prevalence and overlap: a US nationally representative survey. Am J Med 2017;130: 1465.e1-9.
3. Post RE, Dickerson LM. Dizziness: a diagnostic approach. Am Fam Physician 2010;82(4):361–8.
4. Saber Tehrani AS, Coughlan D, Hsieh YH, et al. Rising annual costs of dizziness presentations to U.S. emergency departments. Acad Emerg Med 2013;20: 689–96.

5. Neuhauser HK. The epidemiology of dizziness and vertigo. Handb Clin Neurol 2016;137:67–82.
6. Newman-Toker DE, Edlow JA. TiTrATE: a novel, evidence-based approach to diagnosing acute dizziness vnd Vertigo. Neurol Clin 2015 Aug;33:577–99.
7. Crane BT, Lin FR, Minor LB, et al. Improvement in autophony symptoms after superior canal dehiscence repair. Otol Neurotol 2010;31:140–6.
8. Khalfa S, Dubal S, Veuillet E, et al. Psychometric normalization of a hyperacusis questionnaire. ORL J Otorhinolaryngol Relat Spec 2002;64:436–42.
9. Kerber MD, Kevin A, et al. The Peripheral Vestibular System. In: Baloh and Honrubia's Clinical Neurophysiology of the Vestibular System, Fourth Edition. United Kingdom, Oxford University Press, 2010. p 25-62.
10. Wardlaw JM, Brazzelli M, Chappell FM, et al. ABCD2 score and secondary stroke prevention: meta-analysis and effect per 1,000 patients triaged. Neurology 2015; 85:373–80.
11. Holly LT, Batzdorf U. Chiari malformation and syringomyelia. J Neurosurg Spine 2019;31:619–28.
12. Wall M, George D. Idiopathic intracranial hypertension. Brain 1991;114:155–80.
13. Iljazi A, Ashina H, Lipton RB, et al. Dizziness and vertigo during the prodromal phase and headache phase of migraine: a systematic review and meta-analysis. Cephalalgia 2020;40:1095–103.
14. Lahmann C, Henningsen P, Brandt T, et al. Psychiatric comorbidity and psychosocial impairment among patients with vertigo and dizziness. J Neurol Neurosurg Psychiatry 2015;86:302–8.
15. Shoair OA, Nyandege AN, Slattum PW. Medication-related dizziness in the older adult. Otolaryngol Clin North Am 2011;44:455–71.
16. Strupp M, Brandt T. Vestibular neuritis. Semin Neurol 2009;29:509–19.
17. Kattah JC, Talkad AV, Wang DZ, et al. HINTS to diagnose stroke in the acute vestibular syndrome: three-step bedside oculomotor examination more sensitive than early MRI diffusion-weighted imaging. Stroke 2009;40:3504–10.
18. Dix MR, Hallpike CS. The pathology, symptomatology and diagnosis of certain common disorders of the vestibular system. Ann Otol Rhinol Laryngol 1952;61: 987–1016.
19. Bhattacharyya N, Gubbels SP, Schwartz SR, et al. Clinical practice guideline: benign paroxysmal positional vertigo (update) executive summary. Otolaryngol Head Neck Surg 2017;156:403–16.
20. Epley JM. The canalith repositioning procedure: for treatment of benign paroxysmal positional vertigo. Otolaryngol Head Neck Surg 1992;107:399–404.
21. Yu S, Liu F, Cheng Z, et al. Association between osteoporosis and benign paroxysmal positional vertigo: a systematic review. BMC Neurol 2014;14:110.
22. Hoffman RM, Einstadter D, Kroenke K. Evaluating dizziness. Am J Med 1999;107: 468–78.
23. Whitney SL, Alghwiri A, Alghadir A. fl therapy for persons with vestibular disorders. Curr Opin Neurol 2015 Feb;28(1):61–8.
24. Lanier JB, Mote MB, Clay EC. Evaluation and management of orthostatic hypotension. Am Fam Physician 2011;84:527–36.
25. Newman-Toker DE, Dy FJ, Stanton VA, et al. How often is dizziness from primary cardiovascular disease true vertigo? A systematic review. J Gen Intern Med 2008; 23:2087–94.
26. Staab JP, Eckhardt-Henn A, Horii A, et al. Diagnostic criteria for persistent postural-perceptual dizziness (PPPD): consensus document of the committee

for the classification of vestibular disorders of the Bárány Society. J Vestib Res 2017;27:191–208.

27. Popkirov S, Staab JP, Stone J. Persistent postural-perceptual dizziness (PPPD): a common, characteristic and treatable cause of chronic dizziness. Pract Neurol 2018;18:5–13.

28. Wrisley DM, Sparto PJ, Whitney SL, et al. Cervicogenic dizziness: a review of diagnosis and treatment. J Orthop Sports Phys Ther 2000;30:755–66.

29. Simon NM, Pollack MH, Tuby KS, et al. Dizziness and panic disorder: a review of the association between vestibular dysfunction and anxiety. Ann Clin Psychiatry 1998;10:75–80.

30. Brown JJ, Baloh RW. Persistent mal de debarquement syndrome: a motion-induced subjective disorder of balance. Am J Otolaryngol 1987;8:219–22.

31. Vinik AI, Maser RE, Mitchell BD, et al. Diabetic autonomic neuropathy. Diabetes Care 2003;26(5):1553–79.

32. Black FO, Gianna-Poulin C, Pesznecker SC. Recovery from vestibular ototoxicity. Otol Neurotol 2001;22:662–71.

33. Eibling D. Balance Disorders in Older Adults. Clin Geriatr Med 2018;34:175–81.

34. Parham K, Kuchel GA. A geriatric perspective on benign paroxysmal positional vertigo. J Am Geriatr Soc 2016;64:378–85.

35. Bisdorff AR. Management of vestibular migraine. Ther Adv Neurol Disord 2011;4:183–91.

36. Trinidade A, Goebel JA. Persistent postural-perceptual dizziness-a systematic review of the literature for the balance specialist. Otol Neurotol 2018;39:1291–303.

37. Lopez-Escamez JA, Carey J, Chung WH, et al. Diagnostic criteria for Menière's disease. J Vestib Res 2015;25:1–7.

38. Strupp M, Brandt T. Vestibular neuritis. Adv Otorhinolaryngol 1999;55:111–36.

39. Baloh RW. Clinical practice. Vestibular neuritis. N Engl J Med 2003;348:1027–32.

40. Minor LB, Solomon D, Zinreich JS, et al. Sound- and/or pressure-induced vertigo due to bone dehiscence of the superior semicircular canal. Arch Otolaryngol Head Neck Surg 1998;124:249–58.

41. Eldridge R, Parry D. Vestibular schwannoma (acoustic neuroma). Consensus development conference. Neurosurgery 1992;30:962–4.

42. Lempert T, Olesen J, Furman J, et al. Vestibular migraine: diagnostic criteria. J Vestib Res 2012;22:167–72.

43. Schumacher GA. Demyelinating diseases as a cause for vertigo. Arch Otolaryngol 1967;85:537–8.

44. Thompson AJ, Banwell BL, Barkhof F, et al. Diagnosis of multiple sclerosis: 2017 revisions of the McDonald criteria. Lancet Neurol 2018;17:162–73.

Hoarseness

Hayley Born, MD[a,b], Anaïs Rameau, MD, MPhil[a,b],*

KEYWORDS

- Hoarseness • Voice • Laryngology • Vocal fold • Dysphonia

KEY POINTS

- Hoarseness is a prevalent symptom, especially among professional voice users, such as teachers, and needs to be distinguished from dysphonia, or the clinical observation of disordered voice.
- The differential diagnosis for dysphonia is broad and requires specialized evaluation by an otolaryngologist who can perform office laryngoscopy, preferably with stroboscopy.
- Voice care is multidisciplinary and often requires behavioral intervention by a qualified speech language pathologist.
- Laryngopharyngeal reflux is overdiagnosed and misdiagnosed as a cause of isolated dysphonia, and antireflux medication should not be prescribed without visualization of the larynx.

INTRODUCTION, DEFINITIONS, AND EPIDEMIOLOGY

Voice is produced when the vocal folds (VFs) are set in vibration while adducted through the passage exhaled air, and is modulated by articulation and resonance into human speech. Dysphonia arises with airflow disturbances or when the VF vibratory and/or adductory capacity are impaired. Treatment of dysphonia is targeted toward restoration of normal phonatory function, which requires accurate diagnosis and personalized treatment combining medical, procedural, and/or behavioral interventions. Gold standard clinical care for voice pathologies is multidisciplinary, and involves an otolaryngologist, often fellowship trained in laryngology, and a speech pathologist with expertise in voice evaluation and therapy. Multidisciplinarity is reflected in a joint statement of the American Speech-Language-Hearing Association and American Academy of Otolaryngology–Head and Neck Surgery (AAO-HNS).[1]

Although hoarseness is a symptom referring to the patient's experience of altered voice quality, dysphonia is a sign designating the clinician's observation of impaired voice production or phonation. The distinction of the two terms is primordial, because

[a] Sean Parker Institute for the Voice at Weill Cornell Medicine, New York, NY, USA;
[b] Department of Otolaryngology–Head and Neck Surgery, Weill Cornell Medicine, 240 East 59th Street, New York, NY, USA
* Corresponding author. Sean Parker Institute for the Voice at Weill Cornell Medicine, New York, NY.
E-mail address: anr2783@med.cornell.edu
Twitter: @drhayleyborn (H.B.); @throatbuddha (A.R.)

Med Clin N Am 105 (2021) 917–938
https://doi.org/10.1016/j.mcna.2021.05.012
0025-7125/21/© 2021 Elsevier Inc. All rights reserved.

the experience of hoarseness may not be commensurate to the clinician's observations. Patients may experience hoarseness with no objective findings, or conversely, they may have severe dysphonia with minimal complaints. Hoarseness is assessed with patient-reported outcome measures (PROMs), such as the Voice Handicap Index-10 (VHI-10).[2] Dysphonia evaluation, in contrast, combines the clinician's qualitative assessment of the patient's voice, objective aerodynamic and acoustic analysis, and instrumental examination of the glottis, usually with office laryngoscopy. Dysphonia is distinct from language and speech disorders including aphasia and dysarthria, and fluency disorders, such as stuttering.

Data on the prevalence of voice complaints are limited, and most epidemiologic studies are confined to the North American population. Point prevalence estimates of hoarseness range from 0.98% to 7.6% in the US population, in a treatment-seeking population and a national health survey, respectively.[3,4] The true point prevalence of dysphonia is likely higher, because many patients with voice disorders may not seek medical attention, especially if their voice impairment is temporary and related to an upper respiratory tract infection.[5] Almost one-third of a random sample of adults in Iowa and Utah reported experiencing hoarseness at some point in their lives, and only 5.9% of them sought professional attention from a health care professional or a vocal coach.[6] Prevalence of hoarseness is higher among older adults, with estimates as high as 20% to 29% point prevalence,[7,8] and among females compared with males (1.2% vs 0.7% in a treatment-seeking population).[3]

The portion of the US workforce identified as having high occupational voice use has been estimated to be roughly 20%, including teachers (4.2%) and salespeople (13%).[9] Professional voice users are at increased risk of having dysphonia, especially teachers, among whom estimated point prevalence of hoarseness is 11%.[10] In teachers alone, the cost of hoarseness and associated loss in productivity has been estimated to be in the order of $2 billion annually.[11] Voice problems may account for 72 million lost workdays annually in the United States.[4] Overall, the cost of treating voice disorders is significant, with an estimated $577 to $953 per patient per year, amounting to $13.5 billion per year of potential direct cost.[12]

BACKGROUND
Anatomy of the Larynx

The human larynx functions as a complex musculocartilaginous valve at the junction of the airway and digestive tracts, and is central to several fundamental functions: phonation, airway protection, deglutition, Valsalva maneuver, and cough production. It is made up of the supraglottis, including the epiglottis and ventricular folds (or false VFs); the glottis containing the VFs; and the subglottis, which is the area confined by the cricoid cartilage. It has a bony and cartilaginous framework including the hyoid bone and the thyroid and cricoid cartilages. There are several intrinsic cartilages, the most important being the epiglottis, which aids in airway protection during swallow, and the arytenoid cartilages, which connect to the posterior end of the VFs and facilitate motion. Movement of the larynx as a unit is controlled primarily by extrinsic laryngeal muscles, including the infrahyoid and suprahyoid strap muscles, controlled by the ansa cervicalis nerve (**Fig. 1**).

The intrinsic muscles of the larynx control the refined movements of the VFs in a three-dimensional space. The VFs adduct during phonation and swallow and abduct during breathing and rest. This VF motion is controlled by the action of the recurrent laryngeal nerve (RLN), a branch off the vagus nerve. The RLN arises from the vagus in the upper chest and loops around the aortic arch (ligamentum arteriosum) on the

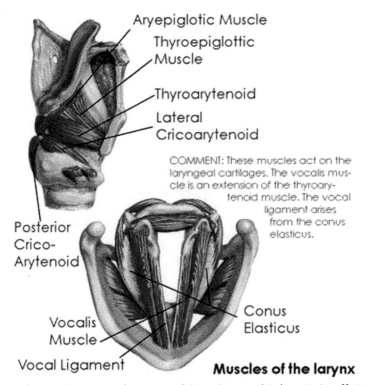

Aryepiglotic Muscle

Thyroepiglottic Muscle

Thyroarytenoid

Lateral Cricoarytenoid

COMMENT: These muscles act on the laryngeal cartilages. The vocalis muscle is an extension of the thyroarytenoid muscle. The vocal ligament arises from the conus elasticus.

Posterior Crico-Arytenoid

Vocalis Muscle

Vocal Ligament

Conus Elasticus

Muscles of the larynx

Fig. 1. Basic laryngeal anatomy. (*From* Noordzij, J. Pieter, and Robert H. Ossoff. "Anatomy and physiology of the larynx." Otolaryngologic Clinics of North America 39.1 (2006): 1-10.)

left and the subclavian artery on the right. It ascends back into the neck in the tracheoesophageal groove to join the superior laryngeal nerve in the larynx. This long, circuitous route makes the RLN susceptible to injury or trauma anywhere along its course. It must be remembered that an immobile VF requires evaluation of the chest and mediastinum in addition to the neck to look for causal factors.[13] The cricothyroid muscle and sensory innervation of the larynx is controlled by the superior laryngeal nerve branch off the vagus nerve.[14]

The VF itself has an intricate anatomy allowing for vibratory sound production. The VFs are anchored at the anterior commissure tendon (Broyles ligament) and the vocal process of the arytenoid. They are composed of three layers: (1) mucosa (epithelium and superficial lamina propria [SLP]), (2) vocal ligament (intermediate and deep lamina propria), and (3) vocalis muscle (thyroarytenoid muscle) (**Fig. 2**). The lamina propria is a triple layer of fibrous tissue with varying densities of elastic and collagenous fibers. The most important of these is the SLP. The SLP, also known as Reinke space, consists of branching, loosely interwoven elastic and collagen fibers underneath the epithelial basement membrane forming an acellular gelatinous layer separated from the intermediate lamina propria by a potential space, Reinke space. This histology allows for fluid-like vibration across the surface of the VF. Many causes of hoarseness are attributed to issues with this layer or the epithelium, which overlies it.[15]

Basic Principles of Phonation

To vocalize, a person must be able to adduct their VFs, build up subglottic pressure (sometimes referred to as breath support), and vibrate their VF tissue. In normal

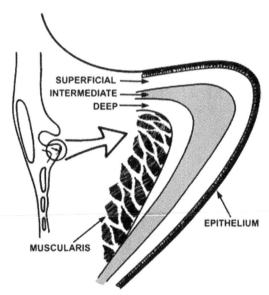

Fig. 2. Histologic anatomy of the vocal fold. (*From* Noordzij, J. Pieter, and Robert H. Ossoff. "Anatomy and physiology of the larynx." Otolaryngologic Clinics of North America 39.1 (2006): 1-10.)

phonation, a coordinated signal from bilateral RLNs causes the VFs to move medially and inferiorly through the contraction of the adductor intrinsic muscles and movement of the arytenoid cartilages. This results in symmetric adduction of the VFs. Pressure then builds up below the glottis by expiration from the lungs. When this pressure reaches a certain threshold, the air escapes through the VFs as they begin to vibrate.[15,16] The vibration propagates across the top of the VF because of the pliability of the SLP and the overlying epithelium. A disturbance in any of these factors may produce a change in voice quality. The inability to adduct and abduct the VFs at appropriate times underlies many of the neurogenic causes of dysphonia. Enough breath support to reach the phonatory threshold pressure is also necessary and may be deficient in pulmonary disorders. Mucosal lesions of the VFs disrupt vibration and therefore also cause dysphonia.

Differential Diagnosis

Causes of dysphonia we discuss here disrupt one or more parts of the phonation process: adduction, subglottic pressure, and/or vibration. One way to categorize pathologies is as inflammatory, neoplastic, neurologic, or muscular. As is often the case, there is overlap between among categories.

Inflammatory

Inflammatory processes that can cause dysphonia include simple inflammation of the VF tissue causing stiffening and disruption in vibrations. This is caused by current or recent viral illness, laryngopharyngeal reflux (LPR), and autoimmune-related inflammation (**Fig. 3**). Postinfectious dysphonia is expected to improve shortly after the illness resolves, as long as continued trauma (coughing/throat clearing) does not persist. An additional infectious cause to consider is laryngeal candidiasis, seen commonly in patients using inhaled steroids.[17,18] An in-depth discussion of reflux

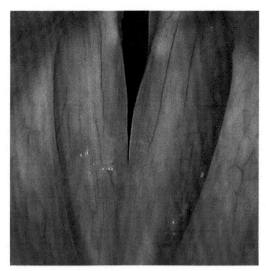

Fig. 3. Reflux laryngitis.

and dysphonia is found later in this article. Importantly, autoimmune and systemic inflammatory diseases can have characteristic effects on the larynx, such as rheumatoid "bamboo" nodules (**Fig. 4**A) or arthritic changes of the arytenoids, amyloid deposits in the VFs, sarcoid granulomas, granulomatosis with polyangiitis changes in the subglottis, and relapsing polychondritis inflammation of the intrinsic cartilages. Systemic lupus erythematosus has also been shown to cause inflammatory changes to the glottis.[19,20]

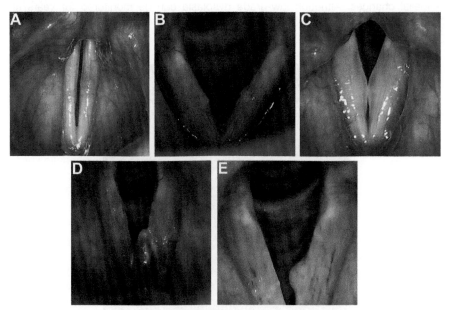

Fig. 4. Benign vocal fold lesions. (*A*) Rheumatoid (bamboo) nodules. (*B*) Phonotraumatic nodules. (*C*) Pseudocyst. (*D*) Polyp. (*E*) Cyst.

Neoplastic

Benign lesions of the VFs are a common cause of dysphonia.[21] Putting aside those lesions caused by systemic diseases, we think of benign neoplastic lesions as phono-traumatic, idiopathic, and viral. Phonotraumatic lesions are benign neoplastic changes that occur at the midfold of the VF, the part of the fold that experiences the most trauma during phonation. A good analogy is to think of a jump rope and how it swings up and down with fixed ends, like a VF. The area where the jump rope hits the ground is analogous to where the VF impacts the contralateral fold. This area is prone to lesion formation, which is chronic (eg, nodules, pseudocysts, polyps, fibrous masses), or acute (hemorrhagic polyps and hemorrhage) (**Fig. 4**B–E). Hemorrhage, although not neoplastic, is phonotraumatic and therefore included here (**Fig. 5**). Naming of these lesions is inconsistent despite attempts to create a clear paradigm.[22] Cysts of the VFs are believed to be congenital or a result of a clogged mucous gland and should be treated with excision to avoid reaccumulation and possible scar.[23]

Another benign neoplastic cause of dysphonia is recurrent respiratory papillomato-sis (RRP), which like anogenital papillomatosis, is caused by the human papilloma vi-rus (HPV) (**Fig. 6**).[24] It can have juvenile and adult presentations. The most common HPV virus strains (6 and 11) in RRP do not typically convert to malignant disease and are also covered by the HPV vaccine.[25] Treatment is not curative and many repeated treatments are expected. It is not yet known what effect widespread HPV vaccination will have on RRP incidence, but it is yet another reason to suggest the vac-cine to patients.[26] In general, treatment or prolonged progression of any of the benign neoplastic VF lesions can lead to scar, a stiffening of the epithelium, or loss of the SLP, which can have devastating long-term vocal effects and these lesions should be eval-uated by a laryngologist.

Many patients present to their primary doctors with hoarseness with concerns for malignant disease. Leukoplakia in the larynx can harbor dysplasia, which is classified after biopsy (**Fig. 7**). Pathologic grades from low to high are given based on features of epithelial changes. Although low-grade dysplasia can be monitored for years for change, high-grade dysplasia and carcinoma in situ are synonymous and warrant

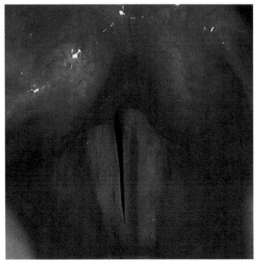

Fig. 5. Hemorrhage.

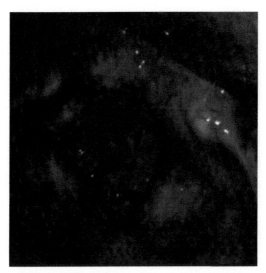

Fig. 6. Recurrent respiratory papillomatosis.

close follow-up with a low threshold for rebiopsy or definitive surgical or radiation treatment. This monitoring should be done in an otolaryngology office using laryngoscopy.[27]

Glottic cancer represents the most dreaded cause of dysphonia for most patients (**Fig. 8**). Although other pathologies exist, squamous cell carcinoma is far and away the most common laryngeal malignancy. It is consistently related to smoking and alcohol use.[28] Treatment paradigms vary based on the extent of the disease and typical staging relies heavily on the extent of invasion into the paraglottic tissues and locoregional lymph node spread. Because of the low blood supply of the glottis, early stage tumors are slow to invade and therefore are able to be treated with

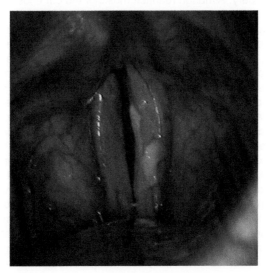

Fig. 7. Leukoplakia.

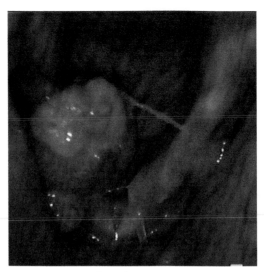

Fig. 8. Laryngeal cancer, squamous cell carcinoma.

conservative excision or radiation. This can preserve function of the glottis and some-times result in return to a near-normal voice.[29]

Neurologic

There are several neurologic pathologies that can affect voice. The most obvious is complete VF paralysis.[30] This refers to the inability of the VF to abduct or adduct because of injury or loss of the RLN. It results in a breathy voice and patients complain about inability to speak without taking frequent breaths. Complete transection may occur iatrogenically in surgeries along the course of the vagus nerve; from injuries at the skull base; to RLN injury in neck surgery (including vascular surgery, cervical spine surgery, and thyroid/parathyroid surgery); and in mediastinal interventions, such as cardiac surgery. Although reanastomosis of the cut ends can be performed, movement is never restored.

Lesser trauma to the nerve, including compression or stretch injury, can happen during surgery or simply because of intubation.[31] These nontransection injuries can result in complete or partial paralysis, known as paresis. VF paresis and paralysis can also occur because of pressure on or invasion of the nerve by malignant disease or even from metastases or lymphadenopathy as commonly seen in patients with lung cancer. Paresis and paralysis can frequently be seen after a viral illness or can be idio-pathic. Any time paralysis or paresis occurs despite an intact nerve there is potential for recovery. The rate and extent of recovery of VF motion depends on the cause of the weakness. Recovery typically happens within 1 year.[32]

All the previous discussion refers to unilateral VF paralysis. Bilateral VF paralysis is much less common and can result from the bilateral occurrence of any of the previ-ously mentioned causes. It results in potentially catastrophic airway compromise and frequently requires tracheostomy. Bilateral VF paralysis is also associated with Chiari malformations and may be a rare manifestation of Lyme disease.[33]

VF paresis is a controversial topic in the laryngology world and has many nuances. Suffice it to say that it is a cause of temporary or prolonged dysphonia in an otherwise normal-appearing patient and is rarely a harbinger of a more serious underlying pathology.[34–36]

There are several other neurologic causes of dysphonia. Tremor, just as it is in the limbs, is a debilitating problem when it occurs in the larynx. Laryngeal tremor is difficult to treat locally; however, systemic treatments are helpful.[37,38] More intriguing is a disease process called spasmodic dysphonia. Spasmodic dysphonia is a rare focal dystonia that results in abnormal speech breaks. It is a result of selective intrinsic muscle hyperfunction. It is predominantly abductor-related or adductor-related, the latter being the most common. It results in a characteristic voice with choppy breaks throughout a sentence in characteristic patterns, and is effectively treated using botulinum toxin injections.[39]

VF atrophy, which can contribute to glottic insufficiency (incomplete closure), is caused by denervation, but it can also be a result of aging. The treatments for VF atrophy are similar to those for unilateral paralysis, so it is included here.[40]

Musculoskeletal

When all other diagnoses have been excluded, there exists a population of patients who continue to have dysphonia. Despite normal laryngeal function, they report hoarse voice, occasionally pain with speaking, and vocal fatigue. These patients may have muscle tension dysphonia.[41] This is a dysphonic state that is the result of misuse of the intrinsic and extrinsic muscles of the larynx. It can persist, similar to a limp, after prolonged compensation for a lesion, or can occur in isolation. As discussed later, careful examination and diligent voice therapy are used to differentiate other pathologies from this.[42]

One final pathology to be discussed is VF fixation. It is an extreme example of laryngeal scarring that results in fusion of the arytenoid to the surrounding tissues. VF fixation can cause dysphonia and airway compromise depending on the extent. It includes unilateral VF fixation, arytenoid dislocation, and posterior glottic stenosis. VF fixation, like VF scar, is difficult to treat. It can be the result of prolonged intubation, malignancy, laryngeal trauma, or iatrogenic injury. VF fixation is an area of active research, innovation, and frustration.[43]

HISTORY

As with all other patient encounters, a full history is vital to characterizing the patient's complaint and narrowing the differential diagnosis. There are several aspects of the history that can guide the diagnostic and treatment approach. One should consider onset, nature, and course of dysphonia, and medical, social, and occupational history.

Onset and timing of symptoms is important to elucidate if the dysphonia represents an acute, gradual, or varying change. If the dysphonia is acute and temporally related to an upper respiratory infection, it is likely to fall into an inflammatory change, that is, laryngitis. A VF hemorrhage or hemorrhagic polyp can result from vigorous cough during these illnesses. Postinfectious RLN weakness or paralysis has also been described. If the onset of symptoms was abrupt after a surgical intervention, such as thoracic, cervical spinal, or thyroid/parathyroid surgery, suspicion for injury to the recurrent nerve and subsequent VF paralysis tops the differential. Postintubation dysphonia may relate to injury to the membranous fold; the arytenoid; or, in the case of prolonged intubation, the RLN or posterior glottis. A longer term gradual onset includes a larger group of the previously mentioned diagnoses but raises suspicion for a neoplastic or neurologic cause. If the dysphonia varies and the patient experiences periods of normal voice, it is unlikely to be a fixed VF lesion. Hoarseness that occurs in the morning or after laying down could direct you toward reflux laryngitis. If the dysphonia is related to voice use, it may relate to a phonotraumatic lesion or a muscle tension dysphonia.

Associated symptoms may help narrow the differential diagnosis. Thin liquid dysphagia is associated with glottic insufficiency because of VF paralysis or atrophy. Shortness of breath while speaking is also indicative of insufficiency from paralysis or paresis. Associated heartburn and regurgitation is suggestive of reflux laryngitis.[44] Weight loss, odynophagia, and hematemesis should raise concern for a malignant disease process, as should ear pain or neck masses.

Medical and social history are extremely important when narrowing the differential diagnosis. There are several systemic diseases that can affect the voice. A history of esophageal dysmotility and severe, uncontrolled reflux might steer the diagnostician toward reflux laryngitis. Autoimmune and inflammatory diseases, such as rheumatoid arthritis, sarcoidosis, lupus, relapsing polychondritis, and granulomatosis with polyangiitis are all known to affect the larynx and subsequently the voice.[19] It is clear that a history of smoking should trigger a complete work-up of persistent dysphonia. Many times this is related to Reinke edema, a characteristic swelling of the VFs SLP related to smoking, but malignancy must be ruled out.[45]

Occupational history is an important consideration in differential diagnosis, and may guide work-up, and referral to otolaryngology. A professional vocalist may notice a subtle change in their voice that has a big impact on their ability to perform and as such complete evaluation should be aggressively pursued. Teachers have a high incidence of dysphonia because of phonotraumatic injuries caused by their high vocal demands.[10]

For a more systematic measure of the severity of dysphonia during history taking, most voice providers turn to PROMs, such as the VHI, the Voice-Related Quality of Life, and their various iterations.[46] These also provide an outcome measure for comparing voice before and after interventions.

EVALUATION OF HOARSENESS
Listening to the Voice

Perceptual assessment of the voice is a fundamental component of the physical examination in patients reporting hoarseness. During history presentation, the clinician should listen for the voice pitch, volume and quality, and intelligibility and rate of speech, and observe posture, respiratory rate, and facial movement. Specific phonatory tasks may be required to reveal subtle anomalies. For instance, the patient may be asked to maintain a sustained/e/after deep inhalation to evaluate maximum phonation time, which is considered abnormal at less than 15 seconds and a possible indication of glottic insufficiency from VF paralysis or atrophy.[47] Other phonatory tasks include changing pitch with a voice glide, altering vocal output with humming, or testing velopharyngeal function (normal with effective soft palate lift and absent hypernasality) with having the patient repeat "ka."

Although perceptual evaluation protocols are often clinician dependent, standardized assessment tools exist. For instance, the Rainbow Passage, an established text including all phonemes of the English language used to elicit speech in individuals with communication disorders, is often read for voice recording to track clinical progress.[48] The GRBAS Voice Rating Scale, developed by the Japanese Society of Logopedics and Phoniatrics, is widely used for perceptual grading of the voice.[49] It uses a four-point rating scale from 0 (normal) to 3 (extreme) for five parameters: G (grade) represents the overall severity of dysphonia, R stands for roughness, B for breathiness, A for asthenia, and S for strain. The Consensus Auditory-Perceptual Evaluation of Voice is another classification system, commonly used by speech language pathologists.[50] Perceptual evaluation helps the clinician formulate a working hypothesis regarding differential diagnosis to be tested with instrumental evaluation.

Laryngeal Examination

The AAO-HNS has issued updated Clinical Practice Guideline for Hoarseness/ Dysphonia in 2018.[5] Among the recommendations is the performance of office laryngoscopy when dysphonia fails to resolve within 4 weeks or irrespective of duration if a serious underlying condition is suspected. Another recommendation is the avoidance of radiologic imaging (computed tomography or MRI) in patients with hoarseness before visualization of the larynx. The duration of 4 weeks was chosen to take into account that most viral laryngitis causing dysphonia, and for which observation is reasonable, resolve spontaneously within 1 to 3 weeks.[51]

Dysphonia persisting beyond 4 weeks is likely caused by pathology that is unlikely to resolve spontaneously, and that requires laryngoscopic visualization for diagnosis. Of primordial concern is delayed diagnosis of laryngeal malignancy or other morbid condition. The AAO-HNS made these specific recommendations with the recognition of the significant delays in referral of patients with dysphonia to otolaryngology, with an average wait between 88 and 119 days.[52] In a survey study, up to 64% of primary care physicians were reluctant to refer patients with chronic dysphonia (>6 weeks) to otolaryngology, preferring initiation of empiric management for gastroesophageal reflux disease (GERD).[53] Earlier referral to otolaryngology leads to more cost-effective therapeutic management compared with treatment without identification of the underlying pathology.[54]

Mirror examination

The traditional laryngeal mirror examination, although it allows for adequate optical resolution of the VFs, has nowadays fallen out of favor because of inability to record the examination and availability of the more advanced techniques of stroboscopy and flexible laryngoscopy. It remains a useful tool in trained hands, and especially in resource-limited settings.

Transnasal flexible laryngoscopy

Transnasal flexible fiberoptic laryngoscopy, available at nearly all general otolaryngology offices, is the most common office laryngoscope used for diagnosis of dysphonia, and is well tolerated by most patients.[55] Its main limitation is the image quality obtained with optical fibers and associated image degradation. The rise of digital image processing in the early twenty-first century led to the miniaturization of charged coupled device cameras and their placement at the distal end of endoscopes, allowing for improved image quality and for affordable single-use flexible laryngoscopes. With transnasal flexible laryngoscopy, the clinician can observe the VFs during connected speech, which is not possible during rigid laryngoscopy with the telescope in the mouth and the tongue retracted.[56] This is particularly helpful in the diagnosis of neurologic disorders affecting the larynx, such as spasmodic dysphonia, vocal tremor, and VF paresis, and the diagnosis of functional laryngeal disorders, such as muscle tension dysphonia or paradoxic VF motion.[57]

Rigid transoral laryngoscopy and stroboscopy

Rigid transoral laryngeal telescopes offer higher-resolution imaging compared with transnasal flexible laryngoscopy, with the transmission of image to the eyepiece via a 70° or 90° lens and a glass rod. It is thus superior in the evaluation of mass lesions and mucosal abnormalities.[58] Combined with stroboscopy, rigid laryngoscopy is the strongest diagnostic instrument in cases of dysphonia caused by a disruption of the normal VF mucosal vibration. Stroboscopy is also available for flexible distal chip laryngoscopes, allowing for pliability evaluation of the mucosal wave via transnasal endoscopy.

Stroboscopy, as opposed to continuous light examination, uses microsecond flashes of light to freeze rapid motion of the VFs to short moments, illuminating different parts of the glottal cycle using light pulses at a slightly different frequency from the VF vibrations. These series of brief images are then synthesized by the retina to a continuous slow-motion vibration of the VFs (**Fig. 9**).[59] Although this technique may be limited in cases of aperiodic vocal pathologies, such as vocal tremor, strobolaryngoscopy remains the single best clinic tool for evaluation of mucosal oscillation abnormalities. It is particularly useful in revealing subtle findings in cases when continuous light laryngoscopy fails to explain the patient's symptom severity.

In the occasional case when office laryngoscopy fails to elucidate the cause of dysphonia, the patient may be taken to the operating room for diagnostic microlaryngoscopy under general anesthesia, to allow for magnified visualization and palpation of the VFs.

Laryngeal Electromyography

Laryngeal electromyography (LEMG) is an important diagnostic tool for determining if VF reduced mobility or complete immobility is caused by paralysis and denervation of the RLN or cricoarytenoid joint fixation. After 10 to 14 days of VF immobility, normal electrical activity on LEMG indicates the latter, whereas patterns of denervation or reinnervation supports the former.[60] LEMG can also be used to detect synkinesis, which occurs after RLN injury with the crossing of adducting and abducting fibers during reinnervation, leading to synchronous contraction of laryngeal muscles that usually have independent neural stimulation.[61] At 4 to 6 months following injury, LEMG has increased accuracy in prognosticating recovery, when dense denervation is more likely to affect intrinsic laryngeal muscles, thus facilitating surgical decision making about VF medialization. Despite its diagnostic value, LEMG is not routinely performed by many laryngologists, likely because of a lack of consensus on methods, interpretation, and validity.

Acoustic and Aerodynamic Analysis

Many multidisciplinary voice clinics complement the diagnostic work-up with sound and airflow measurement of the voice, usually audio recorded by a voice-specialized speech language pathologist. Acoustic and aerodynamic measurements of the voice help identify pathologic voice parameters, determine therapeutic

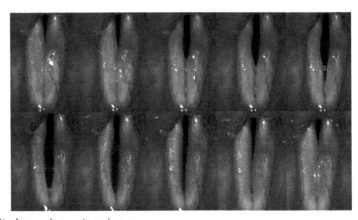

Fig. 9. Stroboscopic montage image.

approaches, and objectify treatment outcomes. Acoustic measures include fundamental frequency (pitch), intensity (loudness), jitter (variations in pitch), shimmer (variations in loudness), noise-to-harmonic ratio, and cepstral peak prominence (degree of organized harmonic structure in connected speech). Aerodynamic assessment quantifies laryngeal airflow and subglottic pressures underpinning voice production.[62]

THERAPEUTIC OPTIONS

Starting with a broad differential and using the history and evaluation techniques described previously, a narrow differential or definitive diagnosis is reached. At this point intervention is directed at the underlying pathophysiology. From least invasive to most, this includes behavioral modifications and voice therapy, pharmacologic treatment, in-office procedures, and surgical interventions. Many times, a combination of these modalities is used.

Behavioral Intervention

Acute inflammation of the VFs after high vocal load or acute infection may resolve with a simple period of relative or complete voice rest.[63] Voice rest is also used during the immediate post-procedural period, although duration and extent varies widely.[64] Voice therapy, however, is an active physical therapy process led by a speech language pathologist. The goals of voice therapy are to optimize healing and prevent recurrence of injury. Voice therapy can also assist patients in optimizing their vocal efficiency in case of permanent injury, such as scar.[17]

Pharmacologic Intervention

Pharmacologic treatment is directed at the underlying pathology. A fungal laryngitis responds well to a course of oral antifungals, just as reflux laryngitis responds to anti-reflux medications, such as histamine blockers and proton pump inhibitors (PPI). Oral, inhaled, and topical steroids have been used in acute inflammation and intraoperatively and postoperatively, although there is controversy as to their effectiveness for uncomplicated laryngitis.[65] Use of the HPV vaccine and local antiviral therapies and immunologic drugs show promise in the treatment of RRP.[66–69] Anxiolytics and β-blockers have been effective in the treatment of vocal tremor.[70] Botulinum toxin injections have been used with great success in patients with spasmodic dysphonia and may help in some cases of vocal tremor.[38,71,72]

In-office Intervention

Botox is a great segue into in-office interventions. Injections of Botox for spasmodic dysphonia occurs in the office of most laryngologists. Many use electromyography guidance. This is extremely well tolerated.[73] Injections for other forms of dysphonia have been on the rise. VF paralysis is treated with an awake, in-office injection medialization using multiple different approaches and materials.[74] It is also useful for patients with other forms of glottic insufficiency, such as atrophy or paresis.[75] Office-based intervention is well tolerated and the indications are broadening every day. Depending on their extent, hemorrhagic polyps, dysplasia, and papillomas can all be adequately treated in the office with laser ablation (**Fig. 10**). Office biopsies and injection of steroids can also be performed. Avoidance of the operating room is ideal in the treatment of dysphonia in patients with comorbidities precluding general anesthesia, individuals requiring frequent retreatments, and those for whom time is a constraint.[76]

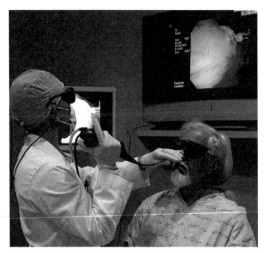

Fig. 10. In-office laser procedure. (*From* Shah, Manish D., and Michael M. Johns M Phila III. "Office-based laryngeal procedures." Office Procedures in Laryngology, An Issue of Otolaryngologic Clinics-E-Book 46.1 (2012): 75.)

Surgical Intervention

When technology, pathology, or patient factors prevent office-based treatment of dysphonia, or when careful dissection is required, such as margins on a malignancy or scar minimization in a vocal performer, microlaryngoscopy is the treatment modality of choice. Using a microscope or endoscopic telescope, precise surgical intervention is taken to treat certain causes of dysphonia.[77] The mainstay of VF surgery is the microflap, which is a precise technique used to minimize scarring.[78,79] Additionally, transcervical, open-neck procedures, such as laryngeal framework surgery or open airway reconstruction, may be needed for optimum long-term treatment of glottic insufficiency, VF paralysis, or airway obstruction.[80,81] New surgical techniques for the treatment of VF scar, laryngeal reinnervation, and other frontiers for the treatment of dysphonia are the subject of several research projects, as the understanding of the pathophysiology of dysphonia deepens.[82–85] New technology using lasers, robotic, and advanced visualization techniques are exciting avenues for innovation.[86–88]

CONTROVERSY: LARYNGOPHARYNGEAL REFLUX
Case Study: Persistent Dysphonia in a Nonsmoker

A 69-year-old male lawyer, with no significant past social or medical history, presented with a 10-week history of hoarseness interfering with his professional demands, treated with a PPI by his internist for the past 2 months with no resolution and worsening voice. The patient self-referred to our clinic. His VHI score was 12/40. His head and neck examination was unremarkable, except for rough dysphonia graded as G1R1B0A1S0. Strobolaryngoscopy revealed a hyperemic lesion involving the left VF at the anterior commissure (**Fig. 11**). An office biopsy was performed, and the pathology report revealed squamous cell carcinoma. This was staged as T1aN0M0 and the patient elected to undergo radiation therapy over surgical excision, and remains free of disease 1 year after diagnosis.

Clinical question: As an internist, would you have managed this patient differently?

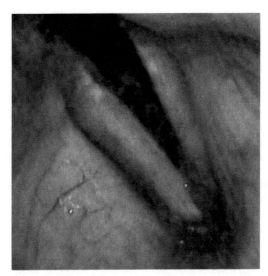

Fig. 11. Case example.

Discussion: Laryngopharyngeal Reflux and Dysphonia

The AAO-HNS 2018 Clinical Practice Guideline for Hoarseness/Dysphonia made a recommendation not to prescribe antireflux medications to treat isolated dysphonia based on symptoms attributed to GERD or LPR, without visualization of the larynx.[5] Many ear, nose, and throat symptoms have been attributed to GERD in the past three decades and have led to the overprescription of empiric PPI even in the absence of concurrent typical GERD symptoms (heartburn and regurgitation). This has led to the overdiagnosis and misdiagnosis of reflux as the cause of the patient's hoarseness complaints, especially among primary care physicians.[53] LPR should not be diagnosed based on the presence of isolated hoarseness without typical GERD symptoms, especially given the limited benefits and possible side effects of PPI. There are no data showing the superiority of PPI compared with placebo in the management of dysphonia, with at least six randomized controlled trials out of nine showing no difference in outcomes.[89–98] As illustrated with the case study, empiric treatment of dysphonia with PPI can result in delayed diagnosis and appropriate treatment.[99]

Additionally, the internal medicine community should be aware that LPR remains a controversial entity within otolaryngology. There are no gold standards for diagnosis either with PROMs, office laryngoscopy, or pH testing, contributing to overdiagnosis and significant cost and safety issues.[100] The cost of LPR care has been estimated to be 5.6 times that of GERD, with pharmaceuticals accounting for 86% of that cost.[101] Empiric management of LPR with PPI has come under scrutiny with growing evidence of potential risks associated with long-term PPI use.[102] Many patients presenting with hoarseness previously attributed to LPR based on fiberoptic laryngoscopy may be found to have other underlying laryngeal pathology on stroboscopy. Suggestive elements of reflux laryngitis on laryngoscopy are not sensitive, and endoscopic findings of VF edema, interarytenoid hyperplasia, or arytenoid erythema thought to be caused by reflux also have been found in normal control subjects.[103,104] There is also no consensus on the type of pH probe, location, or concurrent impedance measurement for the diagnosis of LPR. Mucosal impedance measurement and salivary pepsin assays are still investigational.[105]

DISCUSSION AND FUTURE DIRECTIONS: VOICE CARE IN THE ERA OF TELEHEALTH

In an era of growing telemedicine, patients are increasingly demanding access to laryngology and voice therapy care via virtual means. A decisively limiting factor in the provision of accurate diagnostic evaluation is the current inability to perform remote comprehensive head and neck examination, instrumental evaluation of the larynx, or acoustic and aerodynamic analysis, unless a practitioner with the license and skills is on the patient's side.[106] Currently, telehealth in laryngology is primarily used in prescreening evaluation to risk stratify patients based on symptoms and history and optimize resource use, including clinic visit for laryngeal examination.[107] Conversely, remote voice therapy has been performed for several years to improve access, and has demonstrated cost-effectiveness.[108,109]

With the rapid development of voice recognition technologies, applications of artificial intelligence in the recognition of vocal pathologies have stimulated increasing interest among voice clinicians and researchers, and may help overcome current shortcomings of telehealth. There are existing successful algorithms for the detection of dysphonic voices based on acoustic waveforms and spectrogram automated analysis.[110,111] The main limitation of artificial intelligence diagnosis in dysphonia is the generalizability of models based on small training and validation voice datasets, currently largely limited to single-institution databases. Ensuring diversity in demographics and vocal qualities is also crucial in limiting biased classification by artificial intelligence algorithms.

CLINICS CARE POINTS

- Office laryngoscopy is recommended when dysphonia fails to resolve within 4 weeks or irrespective of duration if a serious underlying condition is suspected.
- Antireflux medications should not be prescribed to treat isolated dysphonia based on symptoms attributed to reflux, without visualization of the larynx.
- Behavioral intervention with voice therapy is an essential component of dysphonia care.
- Many procedures in laryngology are performed in the office nowadays, bypassing the risks of general anesthesia.

DISCLOSURE

Dr H. Born has nothing to disclose. Dr A. Rameau is a cofounder of MyophonX, a wearable device used to restore speech in patients with limited phonation capacity.

REFERENCES

1. Association AS-L-H, American Speech-Language-Hearing Association. The use of voice therapy in the treatment of dysphonia. 2005. https://doi.org/10.1044/policy.tr2005-00158.
2. Rosen CA, Lee AS, Osborne J, et al. Development and validation of the Voice Handicap Index-10. Laryngoscope 2004;114(9):1549–56.
3. Cohen SM, Kim J, Roy N, et al. Prevalence and causes of dysphonia in a large treatment-seeking population. Laryngoscope 2012;122(2):343–8.
4. Bhattacharyya N. The prevalence of voice problems among adults in the United States. Laryngoscope 2014;124(10):2359–62.
5. Stachler RJ, Francis DO, Schwartz SR, et al. Clinical Practice Guideline: hoarseness (dysphonia) (update). Otolaryngol Head Neck Surg 2018;158(1_suppl): S1–42.

6. Roy N, Merrill RM, Gray SD, et al. Voice disorders in the general population: prevalence, risk factors, and occupational impact. Laryngoscope 2005; 115(11):1988–95.

7. Golub JS, Chen P-H, Otto KJ, et al. Prevalence of perceived dysphonia in a geriatric population. J Am Geriatr Soc 2006;54(11):1736–9.

8. Roy N, Stemple J, Merrill RM, et al. Epidemiology of voice disorders in the elderly: preliminary findings. Laryngoscope 2007;117(4):628–33.

9. Titze IR, Lemke J, Montequin D. Populations in the U.S. workforce who rely on voice as a primary tool of trade: a preliminary report. J Voice 1997;11(3):254–9.

10. Roy N, Merrill RM, Thibeault S, et al. Prevalence of voice disorders in teachers and the general population. J Speech Lang Hear Res 2004;47(2):281–93.

11. Verdolini K, Ramig LO. Review: occupational risks for voice problems. Logoped Phoniatr Vocol 2001;26(1):37–46.

12. Cohen SM, Kim J, Roy N, et al. Direct health care costs of laryngeal diseases and disorders. Laryngoscope 2012;122(7):1582–8.

13. Sanders I, Wu BL, Mu L, et al. The innervation of the human larynx. Arch Otolaryngol Head Neck Surg 1993;119(9):934–9.

14. Friedrich G, Lichtenegger R. Surgical anatomy of the larynx. J Voice 1997;11(3): 345–55.

15. Hirano S, Minamiguchi S, Yamashita M, et al. Histologic characterization of human scarred vocal folds. J Voice 2009;23(4):399–407.

16. Perrine BL, Scherer RC, Fulcher LP, et al. Phonation threshold pressure using a 3-mass model of phonation with empirical pressure values. J Acoust Soc Am 2020;147(3):1727.

17. John A, Enderby P, Hughes A. Comparing outcomes of voice therapy: a benchmarking study using the therapy outcome measure. J Voice 2005;19(1):114–23.

18. DelGaudio JM. Steroid inhaler laryngitis. Ann Otol Rhinol Laryngol 2002; 128(6):677.

19. Carruthers DG. Inflammatory diseases and disorders of the larynx. In: Carruthers DG, editor. Diseases of the ear, nose, and throat. (Second Edition). Bristol: Butterworth-Heinemann; 2013. p. 276–84. https://doi.org/10.1016/b978-1-4831-6795-4.50022-1.

20. Systemic and endocrine disorders of the larynx. Clin Laryngol 2015. https://doi.org/10.1055/b-0034-97754.

21. Reder LS, Franco RA. Benign vocal fold lesions. Pract Laryngol 2015;27–44. https://doi.org/10.1201/b19781-4.

22. Rosen CA, Gartner-Schmidt J, Hathaway B, et al. A nomenclature paradigm for benign midmembranous vocal fold lesions. Laryngoscope 2012;122(6): 1335–41.

23. Rutt AL, Sataloff RT. Vocal fold cyst. Ear Nose Throat J 2010;89(4):158.

24. Taliercio S, Cespedes M, Born H, et al. Adult-onset recurrent respiratory papillomatosis: a review of disease pathogenesis and implications for patient counseling. JAMA Otolaryngol Head Neck Surg 2015;141(1):78–83.

25. Ruiz R, Achlatis S, Verma A, et al. Risk factors for adult-onset recurrent respiratory papillomatosis. Laryngoscope 2014;124(10):2338–44.

26. Singh V, Meites E, Klein A. Monitoring public health impact of HPV vaccination on RRP. In: Singh V, Meites E, Klein A, editors. Recurrent respiratory papillomatosis. Cham: Springer; 2018. p. 33–44. https://doi.org/10.1007/978-3-319-63823-2_3.

27. Zeitels SM. Premalignant epithelium and microinvasive cancer of the vocal fold: the evolution of phonomicrosurgical management. Laryngoscope 1995;105(3 Pt 2):1–51.

28. Muscat JE, Wynder EL. Tobacco, alcohol, asbestos, and occupational risk factors for laryngeal cancer. Cancer 1992;69(9):2244–51.

29. Hoffman HT, Porter K, Karnell LH, et al. Laryngeal cancer in the United States: changes in demographics, patterns of care, and survival. Laryngoscope 2006; 116(9 Pt 2 Suppl 111):1–13.

30. Wang H-W, Lu C-C, Chao P-Z, et al. Causes of vocal fold paralysis. Ear Nose Throat J 2020. 145561320965212.

31. Halan B, Matta R, Sandhu K. Postintubation recurrent laryngeal nerve palsy: a review. J Laryngol Voice 2017;7(2):25.

32. Lee D-H, Lee S-Y, Lee M, et al. Natural course of unilateral vocal fold paralysis and optimal timing of permanent treatment. JAMA Otolaryngol Head Neck Surg 2020;146(1):30–5.

33. Joshi A. Bilateral vocal fold paralysis. In: Kapoor NN, Amitabha R, editors. Textbook of laryngology. New Delhi, India: Jaypee Brothers Medical Publishers (P) Ltd; 2018. p. 318. https://doi.org/10.5005/jp/books/13074_34.

34. Wu AP, Sulica L. Diagnosis of vocal fold paresis: current opinion and practice. Laryngoscope 2015;125(4):904–8.

35. Sulica L. Vocal fold paresis: an evolving clinical concept. Curr Otorhinolaryngol Rep 2013;1(3):158–62.

36. Ivey CM. Vocal fold paresis. Otolaryngol Clin North Am 2019;52(4):637–48.

37. Wolraich D, Vasile Marchis-Crisan C, Redding N, et al. Laryngeal tremor: co-occurrence with other movement disorders. ORL J Otorhinolaryngol Relat Spec 2010;72(5):291–4.

38. Nelson RC, Silva Merea V, Tierney WS, et al. Laryngeal botulinum toxin injection for vocal tremor: utility of concurrent strap muscle injection. Laryngoscope 2019; 129(6):1433–7.

39. Lin J, Sadoughi B. Spasmodic dysphonia. Adv Otorhinolaryngol 2020;85:133–43.

40. Sato K. Atrophy of the vocal fold. In: Sato K, editor. Functional histoanatomy of the human larynx. Singapore: Springer; 2018. p. 317–28. https://doi.org/10.1007/978-981-10-5586-7_23.

41. Clary MS, Schneider SL, Courey MS. Muscle tension dysphonia. Laryngology 2014. https://doi.org/10.1055/b-0034-97945.

42. Cherry J. Vocal disorders (phoniatrics): hoarseness and its causes. In: Cherry J, editor. Ear Nose & Throat for Lawyers. (1st edition). London: Routledge-Cavendish; 1997. p. 415–8. https://doi.org/10.4324/9781843143598-110.

43. Gullane PJ, Novak C. Glottic and subglottic stenosis: evaluation and surgical planning. In: Rosen C, Simpson B, editors. Operative Techniques in Laryngology:Berlin & Heidelberg: Springer; 2008. 37–42. https://doi.org/10.1007/978-3-540-68107-6_6.

44. Gooi Z, Ishman SL, Bock JM, et al. Laryngopharyngeal reflux: paradigms for evaluation, diagnosis, and treatment. Ann Otol Rhinol Laryngol 2014;123(10): 677–85.

45. Byeon H, Cha S. Evaluating the effects of smoking on the voice and subjective voice problems using a meta-analysis approach. Sci Rep 2020;10(1):4720.

46. Portone CR, Hapner ER, McGregor L, et al. Correlation of the Voice Handicap Index (VHI) and the Voice-Related Quality of Life Measure (V-RQOL). J Voice 2007;21(6):723–7.

47. Hirano M, Koike Y, von Leden H. Maximum phonation time and air usage during phonation. Folia Phoniatr Logop 1968;20(4):185–201.
48. Fairbanks G. Voice and articulation drillbook. Laryngoscope 1941;51(12):1141.
49. Hirano M. Clinical examination of voice. Springer; 1981.
50. Kempster GB, Gerratt BR, Verdolini Abbott K, et al. Consensus auditory-perceptual evaluation of voice: development of a standardized clinical protocol. Am J Speech Lang Pathol 2009;18(2):124–32.
51. Reveiz L, Cardona AF, Ospina EG. Antibiotics for acute laryngitis in adults. Cochrane Database Syst Rev 2005. https://doi.org/10.1002/14651858.cd004783.pub2.
52. Smith MM, Abrol A, Gardner GM. Assessing delays in laryngeal cancer treatment. Laryngoscope 2016;126(7):1612–5.
53. Ruiz R, Jeswani S, Andrews K, et al. Hoarseness and laryngopharyngeal reflux. JAMA Otolaryngol Head Neck Surg 2014;140(3):192.
54. Cohen SM, Lee H-J, Roy N, et al. Chronicity of voice-related health care utilization in the general medicine community. Otolaryngol Head Neck Surg 2017; 156(4):693–701.
55. Cohen SM, Pitman MJ, Pieter Noordzij J, et al. Evaluation of dysphonic patients by general otolaryngologists. J Voice 2012;26(6):772–8.
56. Eller R, Ginsburg M, Lurie D, et al. Flexible laryngoscopy: a comparison of fiber optic and distal chip technologies. Part 1: vocal fold masses. J Voice 2008; 22(6):746–50.
57. Rosen CA, Blake Simpson C. Operative techniques in laryngology. Springer Science & Business Media; 2008.
58. Sulica L. Laryngoscopy, stroboscopy and other tools for the evaluation of voice disorders. Otolaryngol Clin North Am 2013;46(1):21–30.
59. Woo P. Stroboscopy. Plural Publishing; 2009.
60. Volk GF, Hagen R, Pototschnig C, et al. Laryngeal electromyography: a proposal for guidelines of the European Laryngological Society. Eur Arch Otorhinolaryngol 2012;269(10):2227–45.
61. Blitzer A, Jahn AF, Keidar A. Semon's law revisited: an electromyographic analysis of laryngeal synkinesis. Ann Otol Rhinol Laryngol 1996;105(10):764–9.
62. Dastolfo-Hromack C, Walsh E. Evaluation of neurogenic voice disorders. In: Weissbrod P, Francis D, editors. Neurologic and neurodegenerative diseases of the larynx. Cham: Springer; 2020. p. 53–65. https://doi.org/10.1007/978-3-030-28852-5_5.
63. Ishikawa K, Thibeault S. Voice rest versus exercise: a review of the literature. J Voice 2010;24(4):379–87.
64. Joshi A, Johns MM. Current practices for voice rest recommendations after phonomicrosurgery. Laryngoscope 2018;128(5):1170–5.
65. Amin MR, Achlatis S, Gherson S, et al. The role of oral steroids in the treatment of phonotraumatic vocal fold lesions in women. Otolaryngol Head Neck Surg 2019;160(3):512–8.
66. Papaioannou VA, Arens C. Treatment outcomes of the recurrent respiratory papillomatosis with Gardasil®. Forschung heute – Zukunft morgen; 2018. https://doi.org/10.1055/s-0038-1639761.
67. Creelan BC, Ahmad MU, Kaszuba FJ, et al. Clinical activity of nivolumab for human papilloma virus-related juvenile-onset recurrent respiratory papillomatosis. Oncologist 2019;24(6):829–35.
68. Poetker DM, Patel NJ, Kerschner JE. Cidofovir modulated gene expression in recurrent respiratory papillomatosis. Int J Pediatr Otorhinolaryngol 2008;72(9):1385–92.

69. Lin RJ, Jun Lin R, Rosen CA. Contemporary management of recurrent respiratory papillomatosis in adults. In: Recurrent respiratory papillomatosis. 2018. p. 103–14. https://doi.org/10.1007/978-3-319-63823-2_7.
70. Barkmeier-Kraemer J. Essential vocal tremor. In: Damico J, Ball M, editors. The SAGE encyclopedia of human communication sciences and disorders. Thousand Oaks: SAGE Publications, Inc; 2019. p. 704–6. https://doi.org/10.4135/9781483380810.n235.
71. Gurey LE, Sinclair CF, Blitzer A. A new paradigm for the management of essential vocal tremor with botulinum toxin. Laryngoscope 2013. https://doi.org/10.1002/lary.24073.
72. Reavis C. Botox for spasmodic dysphonia. Brain Life 2018;14(3):6–7.
73. Epstein R, Stygall J, Newman S. Anxiety associated with Botox injections for adductor spasmodic dysphonia. Logoped Phoniatr Vocol 1996;21(3–4):131–6.
74. Cohen S, Brown C. Transcervical vocal fold injection (in-office). J Med Insight 2017. https://doi.org/10.24296/jomi/149.
75. Kelly Z, Patel AK, Klein AM. Evaluating safety of awake, bilateral injection laryngoplasty for bilateral vocal fold atrophy. J Voice 2020. https://doi.org/10.1016/j.jvoice.2020.01.005.
76. Amin M. Office procedures in laryngology. Saunders; 2012.
77. Noorily SH. Laryngoscopy and microlaryngoscopy. In: Atlee JL, Amitabha R, editors. Complications in anesthesia. Philadelphia: W.B. Saunders; 2007. p. 750–2. https://doi.org/10.1016/b978-1-4160-2215-2.50192-7.
78. Courey MS, Gaelyn Garrett C, Ossoff RH. Medial microflap for excision of benign vocal fold lesions. Laryngoscope 1997;107(3):340–4.
79. Hochman II, Zeitels SM. Phonomicrosurgical management of vocal fold polyps: the subepithelial microflap resection technique. J Voice 2000;14(1):112–8. https://doi.org/10.1016/s0892-1997(00)80101-0.
80. Khaund G. Principles of laryngeal framework surgery. In: Kapoor NN, editor. Textbook of laryngology. New Delhi, India: Jaypee Brothers Medical Publishers (P) Ltd; 2018. p. 200. https://doi.org/10.5005/jp/books/13074_19.
81. Young VN, Zullo TG, Rosen CA. Analysis of laryngeal framework surgery: 10-year follow-up to a national survey. Laryngoscope 2010;120(8):1602–8.
82. Mattei A, Boulze C, Santini L, et al. Modified approach of the anterior commissure for transoral cordectomy in case of difficult exposure: a surgical innovation. Eur Arch Otorhinolaryngol 2020;277(1):301–6.
83. Karle WE, Helman SN, Cooper A, et al. Temporalis fascia transplantation for sulcus vocalis and vocal fold scar: long-term outcomes. Ann Otol Rhinol Laryngol 2018;127(4):223–8.
84. Li M, Zheng HL, Chen SC, et al. [Clinical analysis of selective laryngeal reinnervation using upper root of phrenic nerve and hypoglossal nerve branch in the treatment of bilateral vocal fold paralysis]. Zhonghua Er Bi Yan Hou Tou Jing Wai Ke Za Zhi 2020;55(11):1016–21.
85. van Lith-Bijl JT, Desuter GRR. Laryngeal reinnervation: the history and where we stand now. Adv Otorhinolaryngol 2020;85:98–111.
86. Lin RJ, Iakovlev V, Streutker C, et al. Blue light laser results in less vocal fold scarring compared to KTP laser in normal rat vocal folds. Laryngoscope 2020. https://doi.org/10.1002/lary.28892.
87. Chao JR, Goodman J, Fuson A, et al. Hypopharyngeal applications of a new flexible robotic system in otolaryngology. J Robot Surg 2018;12(3):571–4.
88. Patel VA, Goyal N. Using a 4K-3D exoscope for upper airway stimulation surgery: proof-of-concept. Ann Otol Rhinol Laryngol 2020;129(7):695–8.

89. Havas T, Huang S, Levy M, et al. Posterior pharyngolaryngitis: double-blind randomised placebo-controlled trial of proton pump inhibitor therapy. Aust J Otolaryngol 1999;3(3):243.

90. Fass R, Noelck N, Willis Mr, et al. The effect of esomeprazole 20âmg twice daily on acoustic and perception parameters of the voice in laryngopharyngeal reflux. Neurogastroenterol Motil 2010;22(2). 134-e45.

91. Vaezi MF, Richter JE, Richard Stasney C, et al. Treatment of chronic posterior laryngitis with esomeprazole. Laryngoscope 2006;116(2):254–60.

92. El-Serag HB, Lee P, Buchner A, et al. Lansoprazole treatment of patients with chronic idiopathic laryngitis: a placebo-controlled trial. Am J Gastroenterol 2001;96(4):979–83.

93. Noordzij JP, Pieter Noordzij J, Khidr A, et al. Evaluation of omeprazole in the treatment of reflux laryngitis: a prospective, placebo-controlled, randomized, double-blind study. Laryngoscope 2001;111(12):2147–51.

94. Eherer AJ, Habermann W, Hammer HF, et al. Effect of pantoprazole on the course of reflux-associated laryngitis: a placebo-controlled double-blind cross-over study. Scand J Gastroenterol 2003;38(5):462–7.

95. Wo JM, Koopman J, Harrell SP, et al. Double-blind, placebo-controlled trial with single-dose pantoprazole for laryngopharyngeal reflux. Am J Gastroenterol 2006;101(9):1972–8 [quiz: 2169].

96. Reichel O, Dressel H, Wiederänders K, et al. Double-blind, placebo-controlled trial with esomeprazole for symptoms and signs associated with laryngopharyngeal reflux. Otolaryngol Head Neck Surg 2008;139(3):414–20.

97. Lam PKY, Ng ML, Cheung TK, et al. Rabeprazole is effective in treating laryngopharyngeal reflux in a randomized placebo-controlled trial. Clin Gastroenterol Hepatol 2010;8(9):770–6.

98. Steward DL, Wilson KM, Kelly DH, et al. Proton pump inhibitor therapy for chronic laryngo-pharyngitis: a randomized placebo-control trial. Otolaryngol Head Neck Surg 2004;131(4):342–50.

99. Thomas JP, Zubiaur FM. Over-diagnosis of laryngopharyngeal reflux as the cause of hoarseness. Eur Arch Otorhinolaryngol 2013;270(3):995–9.

100. Dhillon VK, Akst LM. How to approach laryngopharyngeal reflux: an otolaryngology perspective. Curr Gastroenterol Rep 2016;18(8):44.

101. Francis DO, Rymer JA, Slaughter JC, et al. High economic burden of caring for patients with suspected extraesophageal reflux. Am J Gastroenterol 2013;108(6):905–11.

102. Brisebois S, Merati A, Giliberto JP. Proton pump inhibitors: review of reported risks and controversies. Laryngoscope Investig Otolaryngol 2018;3(6):457–62.

103. Hicks DM, Ours TM, Abelson TI, et al. The prevalence of hypopharynx findings associated with gastroesophageal reflux in normal volunteers. J Voice 2002;16(4):564–79.

104. Sulica L. Hoarseness misattributed to reflux: sources and patterns of error. Ann Otol Rhinol Laryngol 2014;123(6):442–5.

105. Patel DA, Blanco M, Vaezi MF. Laryngopharyngeal reflux and functional laryngeal disorder: perspective and common practice of the general gastroenterologist. Gastroenterol Hepatol 2018;14(9):512–20.

106. Bryson PC, Benninger MS, Band J, et al. Telemedicine in laryngology: remote evaluation of voice disorders-setup and initial experience. Laryngoscope 2018;128(4):941–3.

107. Strohl MP, Dwyer CD, Ma Y, et al. Implementation of telemedicine in a laryngology practice during the COVID-19 pandemic: lessons learned, experiences shared. J Voice 2020. https://doi.org/10.1016/j.jvoice.2020.06.017.

108. Rangarathnam B, McCullough GH, Pickett H, et al. Telepractice versus in-person delivery of voice therapy for primary muscle tension dysphonia. Am J Speech Lang Pathol 2015;24(3):386–99.

109. Towey MP. Speech therapy telepractice for vocal cord dysfunction (VCD): Main-eCare (Medicaid) cost savings. Int J Telerehabil. 2012;4(1):37–40.

110. Fang S-H, Tsao Y, Hsiao M-J, et al. Detection of pathological voice using cepstrum vectors: a deep learning approach. J Voice 2019;33(5):634–41.

111. Wu H, Soraghan J, Lowit A, et al. Convolutional neural networks for pathological voice detection. Conf Proc IEEE Eng Med Biol Soc 2018;2018:1–4.

Dysphagia and Swallowing Disorders

E. Berryhill McCarty, MA[a], Tiffany N. Chao, MD[b],*

KEYWORDS

- Dysphagia • Swallowing disorders • Aspiration

KEY POINTS

- Dysphagia refers to the impairment of the swallowing mechanism that may result in penetration or aspiration of secretions of food contents into the airway.
- Dysphagia is common in the general population and can be a significant cause of morbidity and mortality, negatively impacting an individual's quality of life, nutritional status, and overall health; in addition, the health care costs and hospitalization rates associated with dysphagia and its complications are significant.
- Dysphagia has a variety of causes and is categorized by location (oropharyngeal or esophageal) and further subcategorized by mechanism (structural or propulsive).
- Assessment and management of dysphagia is dependent on accurate clinical history taking and can be aided by clinical swallowing evaluations conducted by speech and language pathologists.
- Treatment depends on cause but may include swallowing therapy, proton-pump inhibitors, surgery, or in severe cases, permanent bypass of the swallowing mechanism by interventions like nasogastric tubes or percutaneous endoscopic gastrostomy tubes.

INTRODUCTION
Dysphagia and Swallowing Disorders: Definitions

Dysphagia is a symptom of swallowing impairment that can occur if there is a malfunction with any part of the swallowing mechanism. Dysphagia can reduce quality of life, can compromise nutrition, and may result in penetration or aspiration of oropharyngeal secretions or food contents into the airway, compromising ventilation.[1] Penetration involves passage of material into the larynx, but not beyond the true vocal folds. When material passes below the true vocal cords and into the trachea, this is termed aspiration.[2] In most healthy individuals, aspiration results in a cough reflex as the body attempts to prevent the passage of foreign material into the airway.[3] When subglottic

[a] Department of Otolaryngology, University of Pittsburgh, 203 Lothrop Street #500, Pittsburgh, PA 15213, USA; [b] Department of Otolaryngology–Head and Neck Surgery, Hospital of the University of Pennsylvania, 3737 Market Street, 3rd Floor, Philadelphia, PA 19104, USA
* Corresponding author.
E-mail address: tiffany.chao@pennmedicine.upenn.edu

Med Clin N Am 105 (2021) 939–954
https://doi.org/10.1016/j.mcna.2021.05.013
medical.theclinics.com

penetration fails to elicit this cough reflex, this is known as silent aspiration.[2] Other important terms that relate to swallowing disorders include aphagia (the inability to swallow), odynophagia (painful swallowing), and globus sensation or globus pharyngeus (the feeling of foreign body sensation).[1,2,4,5] Dysphagia can often accompany these other sensations (or in some cases be caused by them), but it does not always. Dysphagia is classified by mechanism: structural dysphagia refers to swallowing difficulty caused by too narrow a lumen or overly large food bolus; propulsive (also known as motor) dysphagia results from problems with peristalsis or impaired upper esophageal sphincter (UES) relaxation.[1] It is possible for dysphagia to be a mixed type as well with both structural and propulsive features. Dysphagia is further classified based on location and which phase of the swallowing mechanism is impacted, typically oropharyngeal dysphagia or esophageal dysphagia.[2,5,6]

Prevalence and Cost

Dysphagia is common with approximately 1 million new cases diagnosed annually in the United States[7,8] or 1 in 25 adults, although only a minority seek care for it.[9] Although prevalence is dependent on the age of the patient, the cause, and the method of diagnosis, one report estimated prevalence in the general population around 20%, and dysphagia seems to occur more frequently in women and older individuals.[9,10] Although this article is aimed at evaluation and management of dysphagia in adults, it is worthwhile to briefly note its prevalence in the pediatric population: although less prevalent than in the elderly population, dysphagia is still a common pediatric condition typically resulting from congenital abnormalities like esophageal atresia, esophageal webbing, and systemic conditions like muscular dystrophy. Conditions like cleft palate can prevent proper latching and result in malnutrition and delayed developmental milestones. Although these pediatric conditions are typically caught and corrected early, some congenital conditions like esophageal webbing and muscular dystrophy continue to negatively impact patient health into adulthood.[11]

Given the natural atrophy of the swallowing muscles and changes in mental alertness that often come with aging, symptoms of dysphagia are especially prevalent in the elderly. Some studies suggest that up to 60% of nursing home residents experience dysphagia, and up to half of all Americans over the age of 60 experience some type of swallowing disorder.[12,13] It is a significant cause of mortality, with the Agency for Health Care Policy and Research reporting more than 60,000 deaths resulting from swallowing disorder complications.[14] Aspiration pneumonia is one of the most concerning complications and is one of the leading causes of death in the elderly as well as a significant source of hospital admissions and delayed discharge in the older population.[2,14,15]

Other complications of dysphagia include choking, bronchospasm, chronic malnutrition and weight loss, muscle wasting, and dehydration.[2,15] In surgical patients, particularly patients with head and neck cancer, dysphagia often results in poor wound healing and reduced tolerance to treatments, such as radiation and chemotherapy.[16] It is a primary cause of delayed discharge for patients.[17] Given these complications, dysphagia has significant morbidity. The health care costs associated with the condition and its sequelae are immense. Multiple studies have found that individuals with dysphagia have longer hospital stays, increased rates of hospital readmission, increased mortality within a year of being admitted to the hospital, and increased use of health care services overall.[2,17–20] One estimate for the cost of dysphagia to the US health care system is between $4 and $7 billion annually.[20]

This cost estimate does not take into account indirect costs like the economic impact of patients lost to the workforce as a result of their dysphagic symptoms.[20]

Beyond the health care costs, there are the costs on emotional and mental well-being. Even mild symptoms can have a profoundly negative impact on quality of life.[2] Inability to eat properly may result in feelings of isolation and embarrassment during social gatherings[21]; this is in addition to possible chronic discomfort and bad breath. Many patients with dysphagia report symptoms of depression and inability to enjoy time with others.[22]

PHYSIOLOGY OF SWALLOWING

Disruption or impairment of any phase of the swallowing mechanism can result in symptoms of dysphagia and can result in penetration or aspiration. Swallowing can be divided into distinct phases, although the oral and preoral anticipatory phases are often grouped together[23]:

1. *The preoral anticipatory phase.* In this phase, sensing food through sight, smell, and taste involuntarily stimulates saliva production in anticipation of intake. Saliva, via both mechanical and enzymatic functions, makes chewing and swallowing easier.
2. *Oral preparatory phase.* The second phase of swallowing is voluntary, controlled by the cortex and brainstem, and involves the transformation of food into a bolus via manipulation by the tongue, teeth, and palate. The bolus, a result of food being masticated and mixed with saliva, is primed for transport to the pharynx.
3. *The oral transport phase.* In the transport phase, the food bolus is propelled to the hypopharynx by the tongue. Once it reaches the tonsillar pillars, it triggers the swallow reflex. In a healthy individual, the oral phase lasts about 1 second.
4. *The pharyngeal phase.* This phase is involuntary and initiated by the swallow reflex. It is further divided into 4 subphases: velopharyngeal closure (prevents bolus regurgitation into the nasopharynx), peristaltic contraction of pharyngeal constrictors (propels the food bolus through the pharynx), laryngeal elevation and closure (provides airway protection and prevents aspiration), and UES opening (allowing the bolus to pass from the larynx to esophagus).
5. *The esophageal phase.* In this final phase, the food bolus passes through the UES via peristaltic contractions involuntarily elicited in response to the swallow. This peristalsis clears residue from the pharynx and through the esophagus. When the food enters the esophagus, the lower esophageal sphincter (LES) relaxes and remains relaxed as the bolus passes into the stomach via peristalsis.[1,2,7,23]

Each of these phases can be functionally evaluated to identify which aspect of the swallowing mechanism is impaired and which will assist in diagnosing the cause of dysphagia symptoms.

In evaluating this swallowing mechanism and its pathologic conditions, it is useful to have a general familiarity with the anatomy (**Fig. 1**) and innervation of the oropharynx and esophagus as well as an understanding of the mechanism of peristalsis.

The muscles of the oral cavity and mastication are innervated by the trigeminal (V) and facial (VII) cranial nerves, whereas the pharyngeal muscles are innervated by the glossopharyngeal (IX) and the vagus (X) cranial nerves.[1,23] Innervation of the UES is more complex. The muscles of the UES, primarily the cricopharyngeal muscle and the inferior pharyngeal constrictors, are also innervated by the vagus nerve, but the musculature that facilitates the opening of the UES during swallowing, the suprahyoid (stylohyoid, digastrics, mylohyoid) and thyrohyoid muscles, are innervated by the V, VII, and the hypoglossal (XII) cranial nerves.[1,23] As a result of the tonic contraction

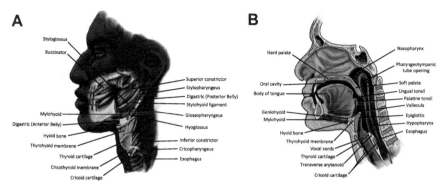

Fig. 1. (A) The musculature of the pharynx and larynx viewed laterally. (B) Sagittal view of the pharynx and larynx. (Acknowledgements: Graphics created by Merriweather McCarty and used with her permission.)

of the cricopharyngeal muscle (by CN X), the UES remains closed at rest. Opening of the UES during swallowing occurs with the relaxation of the cricopharyngeal muscle (brought on by the cessation of vagal excitation) and the simultaneous contraction of the geniohyoid muscle (innervated by C1 fibers traveling along XII) and the suprahyoid muscles (innervated by V), which pull open the UES and displace the larynx forward and upward.[1,23]

When the food bolus passes through the UES, it is moved along the esophagus via peristalsis until it arrives at the LES. Peristaltic contractions elicited in response to the swallowing mechanism are termed *primary peristalsis*; they are the sequential inhibition (called *deglutitive inhibition*) and contraction of the esophageal constrictors, moving the bolus down the length of the esophagus.[1,24] *Secondary peristalsis* is initiated by "bolus-induced distension" of the esophageal wall and can occur anywhere along its length; it begins at the point of distension and proceeds distally.[24] A third type of contraction that can occur in the esophagus is termed *tertiary esophageal contractions*; these are spontaneous, disordered, and nonperistaltic contractions and may lead to impaired acid clearance resulting in gastroesophageal reflux disease (GERD).[25] LES relaxation occurs from the start of deglutitive inhibition until the completion of peristaltic contraction, allowing the food bolus to enter the stomach. At rest, the LES is contracted and closed. The surrounding muscles of the right diaphragmatic crus assist act as an external sphincter during inspiration, cough, and abdominal straining.[1,26] Weakness in diaphragmatic function should be considered as a possible cause or exacerbator of dysphagic symptoms.

Oropharyngeal dysphagia is further separated into 2 categories: oral phase and pharyngeal phase.[2] Oral-phase dysphagia is associated with poor formation of and control of the food bolus. Oral-phase dysphagia typically results in prolonged retention in the oral cavity. It can also be accompanied by drooling, food leakage from the mouth, and difficulty initiating swallowing.[7] The oral phase of the swallowing mechanism (under voluntary control) can be impaired by decreased lip closure, decreased strength in the muscles of mastication, and limited tongue coordination or movement.[7] Pharyngeal-phase dysphagia typically results either from poor propulsion of the bolus by the tongue or via obstruction at the UES. Unlike the oral phase, the pharyngeal phase is under involuntary control, and impairments here may present as delayed swallow reflex, decreased velopharyngeal closure resulting in nasal regurgitation, decreased epiglottic movement and decreased laryngeal elevation on swallowing, or disorders or injury to the UES.[27,28] Depending on the cause of oropharyngeal type, patients may feel globus sensation in the neck or experience nasal regurgitation, aspiration, and symptoms of reflux.[1,27]

Less viscous materials (like water and clear liquids) are more likely to be aspirated in swallowing disorders. Increased substance viscosity slows its transit through the swallowing pathway.[7] Because one of the most common causes of dysphagia is a delayed initiation of the swallowing reflex, this longer time in transit means a greater likelihood that the bolus will be correctly transported.[7]

Esophageal dysphagia can be either structural, propulsive, or mixed in type and can occur in any portion of the esophagus.[13] The esophagus is divided into the cervical portion (from the pharyngoesophageal junction to the suprasternal notch) and the thoracic portion (from the suprasternal notch to the diaphragmatic hiatus).[1] Esophageal dysphagia symptoms are localized to the neck or chest and can include reflux, food impaction, and chest pain. It is important to note, however, that localization in dysphagia is often nonspecific and mixed.[6,13] Management of dysphagia is often dependent on its cause, so accurate diagnosis and understanding of the swallowing mechanism are essential.

CAUSES

As discussed, dysphagia is typically subclassified by location (oropharyngeal vs esophageal) and mechanism (structural vs propulsive). Timing of symptoms, whether they are intermittent or progressive, can help further clarify the cause of swallowing disorders.[1,7,13] **Fig. 2** provides a framework for considering the causes of dysphagia.

Although there is a documented decline in swallowing function with normal aging, more significant symptoms of dysphagia may serve as a herald for further deterioration in health.[2,12,28] Although dysphagia may be caused by a variety of causes, the 2 most common causes result from (1) neurologic or anatomic injury of the cerebral cortex or brainstem and (2) direct injury or damage to the muscles of swallowing.[7] When evaluating patients, it is also important to consider conditions that do not necessarily fit into the framework described above, conditions like chronic obstructive pulmonary disease (COPD), and other respiratory conditions that affect respiration may

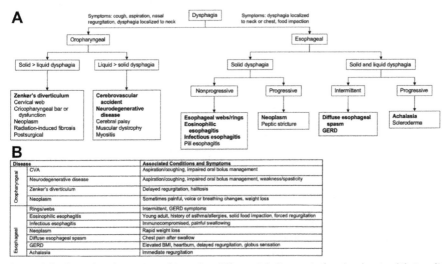

Fig. 2. (A) Algorithm for approaching the differential diagnosis for dysphagia. (B) Conditions in bold represent the most common causes of dysphagia, along with their associated symptoms and conditions. BMI, ; CVA, cerebrovascular accident.

make coordination of respiration and swallowing more difficult and predispose to swallowing disorders.[29]

DISCUSSION
Diagnosis: Differential Diagnosis

An algorithm for approaching differential diagnosis for dysphagia based on symptomology is presented in **Fig. 2**.

Diagnosis: History

Although most causes of dysphagia are benign, symptoms of dysphagia can serve as an early herald for several malignancies and must be thoroughly evaluated. One of the most essential tools in this evaluation is a complete and accurate patient history. Below is a suggested series of questions the generalist should ask to elicit important information:

1. Where does it feel like you have the most difficulty with swallowing?
   - Localization of dysphagia symptoms may point to different causes:
     - Globus sensations localized to the suprasternal notch may point to either oropharyngeal or esophageal dysphagia; more distal dysphagia (esophageal) is referred proximally ~30% of the time.[13,30]
     - Sensations localized to the chest are esophageal in origin 70% of the time.[27,30]
2. How long have you had difficulty swallowing? When do you have problems with swallowing? Is it present all the time or off and on?
   - Timing of symptoms is very important in distinguishing between malignancy and more benign causes of dysphagia:
     - Rapidly progressive over the course of weeks to months may indicate malignancy, especially if it is accompanied by weight loss. Slowly progressive with a background of reflux points toward peptic stricture.[30]
     - Intermittent or episodic dysphagia that has been present for years may indicate a more structural and typically benign process, such as esophageal web or eosinophilic esophagitis.[13,31]
3. What types of food or drinks cause swallowing difficulties? Is it primarily with liquids? Solids? Or both?
   - This may be the most important sign to elicit from your patient.
     - Intermittent dysphagia with solid food only indicates a structural impairment.[32,33]
     - Constant dysphagia with both solids and liquids indicates a motor impairment.[32,33]
4. Do you have any of these other symptoms:
   - *Dry mouth* may contribute to oropharyngeal dysphagia and inability to make a proper bolus from lack of saliva. This symptom might point to an underlying medication issue (**Table 1**) or a systemic problem like Sjogren disease.[34]
   - *Leakage or spillage of food or liquids from mouth* may indicate a problem in the oral phase of swallowing, perhaps a cranial nerve injury.[33]
   - *Nasal regurgitation* indicates oropharyngeal dysphagia and inability to seal off the nasopharynx, or velopharyngeal insufficiency.[33]
   - *Cough, fear of choking with swallowing* may indicate impairment with pharyngeal stage and possible aspiration risk.[2]
   - *Vocal changes and hoarseness*
     - If hoarseness precedes dysphagia, the injury is likely laryngeal and could be a result of chronic damage due to GERD or laryngopharyngeal reflux (LPR).[35]

Table 1 Common medications that can cause symptoms of dysphagia	
Drugs that cause xerostomia (lack of saliva causes impaired food transport)	ACEi: Captopril, lisinopril Antiarrythmics: Disopyramide, mexiletine, procainamide Antiemetics: Meclizine, metoclopromide, ondansetron, prochlorperazine, promethazine Antihistamines/decongestants: chlorpheniramine, cyproheptadine, diphenyhydramine, hydroxyzine, pseudoephedrine Diuretics: Ethacrynic acid SSRIs: Citalopram, fluoxetine, nefazodone, paroxetine, sertraline, venlafaxine TCAs: Amitriptyline, desipramine, imipramine
Anticholinergic/antimuscarinic drugs (lack of saliva and problems with smooth muscle function and coordination)	Atropine, benztropine mesylate, dicyclomine, hyoscyamine, ipratropium, oxybutynin, propantheline, scopolamine, trihexyphenidyl, tolterodine
Neuromuscular blocking agents	Atracurium, cisatracurium, doxacurium, mivacurium, pancuronium, pipecuronium, rocuronium, succinylcholine, tubocurarine, vecuronium
Local anesthetics	Benzocaine, benzonatate, lidocaine
Antipsychotics/neuroleptic medications (pseudo-PD: Tardive dyskinesia can impact patients' ability to chew or swallow)	Chlorpromazine, clozapine, fluphenazine, haloperidol, lithium, loxapine, olanzapine, quetiapine, risperidone, thioridazine, thiothixene, trifluoperazine
Antineoplastics/immunosuppressants (chemotherapy may directly injure esophageal mucosa, predispose to viral and fungal infections)	Azathioprine, carmustine, cyclosporine, daunorubicin, lymphocytic immunoglobulin, paclitaxel, porfimer, vinorelbine
High-dose corticosteroids (skeletal muscle wasting, immunocompromise)	Dexamethasone, methylprednisolone, prednisolone, prednisone
Medications that cause drowsiness or confusion	Antiepileptic drugs, benzodiazepines, narcotics, skeletal muscle relaxants
Medication-induced esophageal injury (pill esophagitis)	Doxycycline, Clindamycin, Tetracycline, Quinidine, aspirin, bisphosphonates, iron, methylxanthines, NSAIDs, KCl, ascorbic acid

Adapted from Balzer KM. Drug-induced Dysphagia, Int J MS Care 2(1):40-50, 2000.[32]

- If hoarseness occurs after dysphagia symptoms have been present, the clinician should be concerned about a compromised recurrent laryngeal nerve, possibly because of advancing malignancy.[1]
  - *Odynophagia or other types of pain on swallowing* typically indicates a type of ulceration that could be caused by infection, inflammatory process, malignancy, mechanical injury, or pill-induced esophagitis.[27,30,32]

○ *Chest pain* may indicate esophageal spasm, achalasia, a peptic stricture if accompanied by reflux, or, more infrequently, an esophageal adenocarcinoma.[30]

○ *Regurgitation between meals or spontaneous regurgitation* at night suggests a dysmotility issue but may also occur with a Zenker or other cervical diverticula.

○ *Reflux*: see Diagnostic Pearl Box 1.

○ *Weight loss*: see Diagnostic Pearl Box 2.

5. What medications are you on?

○ A list of dysphagia-causing medications is provided in **Table 1**. Medication-induced dysphagia is common and can occur with medications that cause dry mouth, impact smooth muscle function and coordination (such as anticholinergics and anti-muscarinics), directly damage mucosa (iron, doxycycline, nonsteroidal anti-inflammatory drugs [NSAIDs]), cause immunocompromise predisposing to fungal and viral esophagitis, or result in decreased awareness, mental functioning, or sensation, especially in the elderly.[13,32] Chronic opioid users are also more likely to present with motor disorders, including esophageal outflow obstruction.[13]

Diagnostic Pearl Box 1: gastroesophageal reflux disease and laryngopharyngeal reflux

One particularly common diagnosis that may lead to symptoms of dysphagia is GERD. GERD can be a cause of dysphagia as well as exacerbate the condition. Chronic reflux may result in anatomic changes, such as strictures, which result in esophageal dysphagia but can also lead to esophageal dysmotility from a variety of mechanisms, including ineffective peristalsis or LES relaxation abnormalities.[35] Other causes of dysphagia, such as achalasia or anything that weakens the UES, may result in symptoms of reflux. LPR shares many pathophysiological mechanisms as GERD but is considered by otolaryngologists to be a distinct condition. LPR is also an inflammatory condition, but it affects the upper aerodigestive tract and involves the reflux of gastroduodenal content, which, like GERD, can result in morphologic changes in these tissues, some which may result in inflammation and cause dysphagia. Reflux episodes in GERD are typically liquid, occur in the recumbent position, and occur at night, whereas reflux episodes in LPR are typically gaseous or less acidic, occur in the upright position, and occur in the day. The 2 may occur together.[36–38] Some studies suggest that LPR may be mediated by factors other than gastric acid, such as pepsin.[39]

Diagnostic Pearl Box 2: Weight Loss and Dysphagia

Dysphagia symptoms alone can certainly cause a significant weight loss, but patients with dysphagia and significant unexpected weight loss must undergo more thorough work-up for malignancy. Regardless of cause, significant weight loss warrants immediate evaluation.

DIAGNOSIS: RISK FACTORS

In addition to the questions listed above, the general practitioner should also elicit information about certain risk factors during their history taking. The presence of certain risk factors may point to 1 cause over another and is useful in diagnosis and management.

Some important risk factors to consider:

○ History of head and neck radiation: results in mucosal injury causing both acute damage and chronic fibrosis, which can result in oral mucositis and weakened musculature of swallowing.[40]

- o Personal or family history of thyroid issues: severely enlarged thyroid or goiter may cause compressive symptoms resulting in dysphagia or globus sensation.[41]
- o History of inflammatory bowel disease (IBD) or celiac disease: oral manifestations and esophageal lesions associated with IBD may cause dysphagia symptoms.[42] Patients with celiac disease may also present with esophageal webs that cause dysphagia.[43]
- o History of prolonged intubation, esophageal or head and neck surgery, or ingestion of caustic material or pills may predispose to strictures.[32,44,45]
- o History of atopy or allergy may point toward eosinophilic esophagitis.[46]
- o Current use of chemotherapy or diagnosis of an immunocompromised state like HIV/AIDS should alert the clinician to the possibility of esophagitis owing to opportunistic infections like Candida, herpes simplex virus, cytomegalovirus (CMV), or tumors like Kaposi sarcoma or lymphoma.[47]
- o History of recurrent pneumonia or chest infections may indicate presence of silent aspiration.[2]

DIAGNOSIS: PHYSICAL EXAMINATION

Once a complete patient history has been collected, a targeted physical examination should be completed. It is important to note here that dysphagia is often only 1 manifestation of more systemic disease processes, particularly of muscular dystrophies, conditions like scleroderma, or other neuromuscular and connective tissue diseases. In evaluating oropharyngeal dysphagia, clinicians should look for the following signs:

- *Neuromuscular conditions:* Dysarthria, dysphonia, ptosis, tongue atrophy.[33]
- *Neck:* Examine for thyromegaly or other masses; presence of Virchow node in the left supraclavicular fossa is associated with esophageal cancer.[33,40]
- *Mouth and pharynx:* Examine dentition (absent or poor dentition can interfere with mastication), check for buccal lesions and ulcerations, and look for signs of opportunistic infection.[33]
- *Skin:* Certain rashes may suggest diagnosis of scleroderma or mucocutaneous conditions that can affect the esophagus.[48–50]
- *Respiratory:* Cough, wheezing, desaturations may indicate either current silent aspiration pneumonia or a respiratory cause like COPD.[29]

Physical examination is less helpful in evaluating esophageal dysphagia given the difficulty of examining the larynx and esophagus in the typical general internist's clinic. If the physical examination is unrevealing and the patient is suspected of having esophageal dysphagia, the next recommended step is referral to an otolaryngologist or gastroenterology for more advanced examination techniques. If a neurologic cause is suspected, a complete neurologic workup is recommended.

DIAGNOSIS: ADVANCED TECHNIQUES

Details of the history and initial physical examination will guide the next steps in diagnosis. More advanced diagnostic procedures can be conducted by gastroenterologists, radiologists, otolaryngologists, or speech and language pathologists (SLPs) depending on reported symptoms. An otolaryngologist may perform a flexible fiberoptic laryngoscopic examination of the nasopharynx, oropharynx, hypopharynx, and larynx to assess for masses, mucosal lesions, pooling of secretions, or other structural issues. If oropharyngeal dysphagia is suspected based on history and physical examination, the patient should be referred to a health care professional who is trained to conduct a clinical swallowing examination (CSE), typically an SLP. This test provides additional information about the patient's cognition, phonation, functionality of the cranial nerves involved in swallowing, speech intelligibility, and cough strength to examine how well the patient handles secretions. This test also typically assesses swallowing with foods and liquids of different consistencies.[7,33] Following a CSE, a fiberoptic endoscopic evaluation of swallowing (FEES) study may be performed. FEES should be used if there is a concern for silent aspiration or motility issues. It involves the use of a flexible fiberoptic laryngoscope to visualize the larynx and pharynx and evaluate swallowing mechanism and management of secretions, typically while the patient swallows different consistencies of liquids or solids that have been colored with a food dye for improved visualization of the material.[7,28,51] An FEES can be performed at the bedside, but is limited by a brief "white-out" phase during the swallow itself, precluding direct examination of the swallowing mechanism. Information is obtained from observation of pharyngeal sensation and location of the bolus before and after the swallow.

A modified barium swallow study (MBSS), also known as a videofluoroscopic swallowing study, can also be used to evaluate the oral and pharyngeal phases of swallowing and provides dynamic information on the oropharyngeal and pharyngoesophageal phases of swallowing. Similar to a CSE, in an MBSS, the patient is observed eating a variety of foods at different consistencies, but unlike a CSE, the food is coated with barium, and the patient is seated in front of an X-ray or fluoroscopy machine that allows for visualization of the swallowing mechanism and peristalsis. Unlike FEES, this test allows for real-time visualization of pharyngeal and esophageal muscle contraction and relaxation and can also detect minute amounts of aspiration or penetration.[7,52] In addition, it is possible to measure temporal characteristics of swallowing, such as transit time. MBSS includes the need for specialized equipment, which requires both a radiologist and an SLP, and like an esophagram, it requires exposure to radiation, making it unsuitable for pregnant women or multiple re-testings, unlike FEES.[7,52,53] Although an MBSS can detect gross structural abnormalities of the oropharynx and esophagus, it is designed to provide information on swallowing function and should not be used as an initial diagnostic tool if a structural cause of dysphagia is more likely and there is no concern for aspiration.

If esophageal dysphagia is suspected, 2 different procedures are typically used as an initial diagnostic workup: upper endoscopy (esophagoscopy) and a barium swallow study (esophagram). In evaluating esophageal dysphagia, flexible esophagoscopy may be the single most useful procedure. It provides better visualization of mucosal lesions and masses than an esophagram or MBSS, and it allows for direct mucosal biopsies.[54] In addition, esophagoscopy allows for immediate therapeutic intervention with esophageal dilation if needed. The more recent emergence of eosinophilic esophagitis as a cause of unexplained dysphagia has led to the recommendation that mucosal biopsies be routinely obtained even if mucosal lesions are absent.[55] Esophagoscopy is typically performed under anesthesia by a gastroenterologist, but some otolaryngologists are able to perform awake transnasal esophagoscopy in the office.[56]

An esophagram (barium swallow) evaluates the entire esophagus and can be used in addition to esophagoscopy for visualization of possible structural causes of dysphagia. However, a barium swallow should be performed before endoscopy if a proximal esophageal lesion is suspected or if there is a history or clinical suspicion for stricture. The patient drinks a barium liquid and is seated in front of an X-ray or fluoroscopy machine that allows for visualization of the esophagus during liquid transit. It only requires a radiologist and can provide additional information about possible masses, strictures, esophageal dysmotility, and abnormalities like hiatal hernias and Zenker diverticulum. An esophagram is typically done if the dysphagia is not adequately explained by endoscopy or additional information is needed.[53] Patients

Table 2
Diagnostic techniques to evaluate dysphagia

Diagnostic Technique	Description	Useful for	Disadvantages
CSE	Comprehensive bedside evaluation by SLP	Patients with concern for aspiration or other functional swallowing disturbances	Does not provide comprehensive structural information
FEES	Flexible fiberoptic pharyngolaryngoscopic examination performed while patient swallows foods and liquids of various consistencies	Detection of structural or sensory abnormalities in the oropharynx, hypopharynx, or larynx; assessment of aspiration or penetration; can be performed at bedside	Unable to directly view pharyngeal structures during active phase of swallowing
Flexible esophagoscopy	Flexible fiberoptic evaluation of esophagus	Structural evaluation of esophagus, can perform biopsies	Typically performed under anesthesia; poor visualization of pharynx and region around UES
Rigid esophagoscopy	Rigid transoral evaluation of oropharynx, hypopharynx, and upper esophagus	Structural evaluation of pharynx and upper esophagus, can perform biopsies	Requires general anesthesia, unable to evaluate distal esophagus in adults
Esophagram (barium swallow)	Video fluoroscopic study used to evaluate esophageal contour and transit of barium liquid or pill	Structural evaluation of esophagus, also provides some information on esophageal motility	Radiation exposure
Modified barium swallowing study (MBSS)	Video fluoroscopic evaluation of swallowing performed with speech language pathologist	Detection of dysfunctional swallow in oral, oropharyngeal, and esophageal phases; gross pharyngeal or esophageal structural abnormalities	Radiation exposure
24-h pH monitoring	Placement of transnasal flexible catheter to detect reflux events	Gold standard for detection of GERD, dual channel probes may detect LPR, and addition of impedance probes may detect nonacid reflux events	Patient discomfort from presence of transnasal catheter for 24 h
High-resolution manometry	Pressure-sensing catheter placed transnasally	Detection of esophageal dysmotility or abnormalities of UES and LES	

with otherwise negative workups on barium swallow and endoscopy may undergo high-resolution esophageal manometry to determine whether a motility disorder is present.

Although these diagnostic techniques are perhaps the most commonly used in the evaluation of dysphagia, there is currently no standardized protocol for dysphagia screening, and different institutions may follow their own guidelines.[57] There are a variety of other diagnostic techniques that may also be used; a brief list and description of them are included in **Table 2**.

MANAGEMENT

Treatment of dysphagia is highly dependent on cause. If the dysphagia is part of a systemic condition like a neuromuscular disease or an autoimmune disease, the most effective management is treatment of the underlying condition. For oropharyngeal dysphagia resulting from functional deficits, the primary aim in management should be on educating the patient on how to eat safely and reduce aspiration risk. If a medication is causing the symptoms, recommendations are to switch medications, and if that is not possible, then to engage in swallowing therapy. The SLPs serve an important role here and can teach patients swallowing exercises and safer positions to eat in that will protect the lungs; this is particularly useful after cerebrovascular accidents or other neurologic events. In addition, diet changes are usually recommended after a CSE, only allowing foods of a certain viscosity. This type of dietary modification has been shown to reduce risk of aspiration pneumonia. In many cases, the functional swallowing deficits caused by stroke will resolve over time, but if they do not, then it may be appropriate to consider a nasogastric tube or gastrostomy with enteral feedings. Non-oral feeding methods should also be considered for progressive neurologic conditions like amyotrophic lateral sclerosis and Parkinson disease (PD), although these patients are still at risk of aspirating salivary secretions. Surgical procedures, such as laryngeal suspension and vocal cord augmentation, may also be used to reduce aspiration risk.[30] Myotomy (diverticulotomy) via open surgical or endoscopic approach is appropriate for cricopharyngeal bars or Zenker diverticulum.[58]

Structural esophageal dysphagia resulting from neoplasm or achalasia can also be surgically managed, or endoscopic dilatation may be done as a palliative measure to improve quality of life. In the case of strictures or other structural esophageal dysphagia, endoscopic dilatation via bougie or a balloon dilator is often effective management; if severe, myotomy is also an option.[13] If the cause of esophageal dysphagia is infection, such as CMV or candida, it is best to treat the underlying infection and consider antibiotic, antiviral, or antifungal prophylaxis in the case of immunocompromised patients. Eosinophilic esophagitis can be effectively treated by elimination diet and proton-pump inhibitors (PPI); swallowed topical steroids can be given in severe cases, and dilation can be used if strictures have developed.[59]

In almost all cases though, management of dysphagia is multidisciplinary, involving clinicians, SLPs, and dieticians. Patients should be educated on how to eat safely; diet should be optimized, and PPIs or other acid suppression medications should be used, especially in the case of GERD or LPR.[13] Empiric dilation in combination with PPI, even in the absence of stricture or in the presence of mild strictures, is common in clinical management,[60] although other studies dispute such practice.[61]

SUMMARY

Dysphagia, defined as impairment of the swallowing process, is a common symptom and is a significant source of morbidity and mortality in the general population. Not only are the health care costs associated with dysphagia and its complications immense, but also swallowing disorders dramatically alter the quality of life of the unfortunate patients who suffer from them, negatively impacting their ability to socialize with loved ones or enjoy a meal. Dysphagia has a variety of causes, and elucidating the correct cause is essential in management of the condition. Broadly, dysphagia can be classified as oropharyngeal or esophageal and structural or propulsive. A multidisciplinary approach is typically required for effective diagnosis and treatment and may involve neurologists, radiologists, otolaryngologists, and SLPs. Treatment is dependent on cause and ranges from medical management of associated symptoms to swallowing therapy to surgery. It is a fascinating symptom that demands a clinician with deft history-taking skills and a thorough knowledge of the pathophysiology of swallowing.

CLINICS CARE POINTS

- A detailed and complete medical history is the single most important diagnostic tool in the diagnosis and management of dysphagia. It is necessary for distinguishing oropharyngeal dysphagia from esophageal dysphagia, a determination that will direct next steps in care.
- Recurrent pneumonias (especially if they are localized to the lower right lobe) may indicate the presence of silent aspiration and warrant a complete swallowing evaluation.
- Although symptoms of dysphagia alone can cause a significant weight loss, rapid and unexpected weight loss is an alarm symptom and warrants immediate and thorough evaluation for possible malignancy.
- Not only are speech and language pathologists helpful in the diagnosis of swallowing disorders but also they are often essential in the treatment of dysphagia; they train patients in safe swallowing technique, guide dietary modifications, and continue to be an active part of a patient's swallowing therapy. Their role highlights the multidisciplinary nature in the management and treatment of swallowing disorders.
- The 3 most common and useful advanced techniques in the diagnosis of dysphagia are fiberoptic endoscopic evaluation of swallowing, modified barium swallow, and esophagoscopy.
- Management of dysphagia is dependent on cause and may include treatment of an underlying condition, acid suppression medication, endoscopic dilation of the esophagus, surgery, diet modification, swallowing therapy, or some combination of these treatments.

DISCLOSURE

The authors have no commercial or financial conflicts to disclose.

REFERENCES

1. Hirano I, Kahrilas P. Chapter 53: dysphagia. In: Kasper DL, Hauser SL, Jameson JL, et al, editors. Harrison's principles of internal medicine, 19th edition. Basic principles and cardinal manifestations of disease, vol. 1. McGraw-Hill Education; 2018. p. 254–8.
2. Lancaster J. Dysphagia: its nature, assessment and management. Br J Community Nurs 2015;Suppl Nutrition:S28–32.
3. Davenport PW. Urge-to-cough: what can it teach us about cough? Lung 2008; 186(Suppl 1):S107–11.

4. Lee BE, Kim GH. Globus pharyngeus: a review of its etiology, diagnosis and treatment. World J Gastroenterol 2012;18(20):2462–71.
5. Triggs J, Pandolfino J. Recent advances in dysphagia management [version 1; peer review: 3 approved]. F1000Research 2019;8(F1000 Faculty Rev):1527.
6. Roeder BE, Murray JA, Dierkhising RA. Patient localization of esophageal dysphagia. Dig Dis Sci 2004;49(4):697–701.
7. Treviso-Jones L, Skidmore K. Chapter 74: dysphagia and aspiration.. In: Scholes MA, Ramakrishnan VR, editors. ENT secrets. 4th edition. Philadelphia: Elsevier Health Sciences; 2015. p. 507–13.
8. Encore Medical, L.P. -4599A 0505 "Dysphagia Fact Sheet" from Vital Care Tech. Available at: https://www.djoglobal.com/sites/default/files/vitalstim/Dysphagia%20fact%20sheet.pdf. Accessed October 15, 2020.
9. Bhattacharyya N. The prevalence of dysphagia among adults in the United States. Otolaryngol Head Neck Surg 2014;151(5):765–9.
10. Wilkins T, Gillies RA, Thomas AM, et al. The prevalence of dysphagia in primary care patients: a HamesNet Research Network study. J Am Board Fam Med 2007;20:144–50.
11. Dodrill P, Gosa M. Pediatric dysphagia: physiology, assessment, and management. Ann Nutr Metab 2015;66:24–31.
12. Baijens LW, Clavé P, Cras P, et al. European Society for Swallowing Disorders - European Union Geriatric Medicine Society white paper: oropharyngeal dysphagia as a geriatric syndrome. Clin Interv Aging 2016;11:1403–28.
13. Johnston BT. Oesophageal dysphagia: a stepwise approach to diagnosis and management. Lancet Gastroenterol Hepatol 2017;2(8):604–9.
14. American Speech-Language-Hearing Association. Adult dysphagia. (practice portal). Available at: www.asha.org/Practice-Portal/Clinical-Topics/Adult-Dysphagia/. Accessed November 10, 2020.
15. Mandell LA, Niederman MS. Aspiration pneumonia. N Engl J Med 2019;380(7):651–63.
16. Gaziano JE. Evaluation and management of oropharyngeal dysphagia in head and neck cancer. Cancer Control 2002;9(5):400–9.
17. Maeshima S, Osawa A, Miyazaki Y, et al. Influence of dysphagia on short-term outcome in patients with acute stroke. Am J Phys Med Rehabil 2011;90(4):316–20.
18. Jukic Peladic N, Orlandoni P, Dell'Aquila G, et al. Dysphagia in nursing home residents: management and outcomes. J Am Med Dir Assoc 2019;20(2):147–51.
19. Attrill S, White S, Murray J, et al. Impact of oropharyngeal dysphagia on healthcare cost and length of stay in hospital: a systematic review. BMC Health Serv Res 2018;18(1):594.
20. Patel DA, Krishnaswami S, Steger E, et al. Economic and survival burden of dysphagia among inpatients in the United States. Dis Esophagus 2018;31(1):1–7.
21. Ekberg O, Hamdy S, Woisard V, et al. Social and psychological burden of dysphagia: its impact on diagnosis and treatment. Dysphagia 2002;17:139–46.
22. Farri A, Accornero A, Burdese C. Social importance of dysphagia: its impact on diagnosis and therapy. Acta Otorhinolaryngol Ital 2007;27(2):83–6.
23. Matsuo K, Palmer JB. Anatomy and physiology of feeding and swallowing: normal and abnormal. Phys Med Rehabil Clin N Am 2008;19(4):691–vii.
24. Nikaki K, Sawada A, Ustaoglu A, et al. Neuronal control of esophageal peristalsis and its role in esophageal disease. Curr Gastroenterol 2019;21:59.
25. Triadafilopoulos G, Castillo T. Nonpropulsive esophageal contractions and gastroesophageal reflux. Am J Gastroenterol 1991;86(2):153–9.

26. Mittal RK, Kumar D, Kligerman SJ, et al. Three-dimensional pressure profile of the lower esophageal sphincter and crural diaphragm in patients with achalasia esophagus. Gastroenterology 2020;159(3):864–72.e1.
27. Clavé P, Shaker R. Dysphagia: current reality and scope of the problem. Nat Rev Gastroenterol Hepatol 2015;12:259–70.
28. Cook IJ. Oropharyngeal dysphagia. Gastroenterol Clin North Am 2009;38(3): 411–31.
29. Ghannouchi I, Speyer R, Doma K, et al. Swallowing function and chronic respiratory diseases: systematic review. Respir Med 2016;117:54–64.
30. Cook IJ. Diagnostic evaluation of dysphagia. Nat Clin Pract Gastroenterol Hepatol 2008;5(7):393–403.
31. Lee GS, Craig PI, Freiman JS, et al. Intermittent dysphagia for solids associated with a multiringed esophagus: clinical features and response to dilatation. Dysphagia 2007;22(1):55–62.
32. Balzer KM. Drug-induced dysphagia. Int J MS Care 2000;2(1):40–50.
33. Abdel Jalil AA, Katzka DA, Castell DO. Approach to the patient with dysphagia. Am J Med 2015;128(10). 1138.e17-1138.e1.138E23.
34. Napeñas JJ, Rouleau TS. Oral complications of Sjögren's syndrome. Oral Maxillofac Surg Clin North Am 2014;26(1):55–62.
35. Martinucci I, de Bortoli N, Giacchino M, et al. Esophageal motility abnormalities in gastroesophageal reflux disease. World J Gastrointest Pharmacol Ther 2014; 5(2):86–96.
36. Postma GN, Halum SL. Laryngeal and pharyngeal complications of gastroesophageal reflux disease. GI Motil Online 2006.
37. Lechien JR, Bobin F, Muls V, et al. Gastroesophageal reflux in laryngopharyngeal reflux patients: clinical features and therapeutic response. Laryngoscope 2020; 130:E479–89.
38. Koufman JA. Laryngopharyngeal reflux is different from classic gastroesophageal reflux disease. Ear Nose Throat J 2002;81(suppl 2):7–9.
39. Pearson JP, Parikh S. Review article: nature and properties of gastro-oesophageal and extra-oesophageal refluxate. Aliment Pharmacol Ther 2011; 33(Suppl. 1):1–71.
40. King SN, Dunlap NE, Tennant PA, et al. Pathophysiology of radiation-induced dysphagia in head and neck cancer. Dysphagia 2016;31:339–51.
41. Sorensen JR, Bonnema SJ, Godballe C, et al. The impact of goiter and thyroid surgery on goiter related esophageal dysfunction. A systematic review. Front Endocrinol (Lausanne) 2018;9:679.
42. Lauritano D, Boccalari E, Di Stasio D, et al. Prevalence of oral lesions and correlation with intestinal symptoms of inflammatory bowel disease: a systematic review. Diagnostics (Basel) 2019;9(3):77.
43. Sinha SK, Nain CK, Udawat HP, et al. Cervical esophageal web and celiac disease. J Gastroenterol Hepatol 2008;23(7 Pt 1):1149–52.
44. Brodsky MB, Huang M, Shanholtz C, et al. Recovery from dysphagia symptoms after oral endotracheal intubation in acute respiratory distress syndrome survivors: a 5-year longitudinal study. Ann Am Thorac Soc 2017;14:376–83.
45. Messing BP, Ward EC, Lazarus C, et al. Establishing a multidisciplinary head and neck clinical pathway: an implementation evaluation and audit of dysphagia-related services and outcomes. Dysphagia 2019;34(1):89–104.
46. Gómez-Aldana A, Jaramillo-Santos M, Delgado A, et al. Eosinophilic esophagitis: current concepts in diagnosis and treatment. World J Gastroenterol 2019;25(32): 4598–613.

47. Raufman JP. Odynophagia/dysphagia in AIDS. Gastroenterol Clin North Am 1988;17(3):599–614.
48. Fulp SR, Castell DO. Scleroderma esophagus. Dysphagia 1990;5(4):204–10.
49. Irisarri Garde R, Borobio Aguilar E, Cebrián García A. Esophageal lichen planus: a rare cause of dysphagia. Rev Esp Enferm Dig 2019;111(8):652.
50. Zehou O, Raynaud JJ, Le Roux-Villet C, et al. Oesophageal involvement in 26 consecutive patients with mucous membrane pemphigoid. Br J Dermatol 2017; 177(4):1074–85.
51. Bours Speyer R, Lemmens J, Limburg M, et al. Bedside screening tests vs. videofluoroscopy or fibreoptic endoscopic evaluation of swallowing to detect dysphagia in patients with neurological disorders: systematic review. J Adv Nurs 2009;65(3):477–93.
52. Hazelwood RJ, Armeson KE, Hill EG, et al. Identification of swallowing tasks from a modified barium swallow study that optimize the detection of physiological impairment. J Speech Lang Hear Res 2017;60(7):1855–63.
53. Birzes K. Clarification between an MBS and esophagram. Wellspan Imaging Reference Guide. 2012. Available at: https://www.wellspan.org/media/4111/mbs-vs-esophagram-r3-28-2012.pdf. Accessed November 10, 2020.
54. Levine B, Nielsen EW. The justifications and controversies of panendoscopy—a review. Ear Nose Throat J 1992;71(8):335–40, 343.
55. Ricker J, McNear S, Cassidy T, et al. Routine screening for eosinophilic esophagitis in patients presenting with dysphagia. Therap Adv Gastroenterol 2011;4(1): 27–35.
56. Postma GN, Cohen JT, Belafsky PC, et al. Transnasal esophagoscopy: revisited (over 700 consecutive cases). Laryngoscope 2005;115(2):321–3.
57. Daniels SK, Anderson JA, Willson PC. Valid items for screening dysphagia risk in patients with stroke: a systematic review. Stroke 2012;43(3):892–7.
58. Bizzotto A, Iacopini F, Landi R, et al. Zenker's diverticulum: exploring treatment options. Acta Otorhinolaryngol Ital 2013;33(4):219–29.
59. Shah NA, Albert DM, Hall NM, et al. Managing eosinophilic esophagitis: challenges and solutions. Clin Exp Gastroenterol 2016;9:281–90.
60. Olson JS, Lieberman DA, Sonnenberg A. Empiric dilation in non-obstructive dysphagia. Dig Dis Sci 2008;53(5):1192–7.
61. Lavu K, Mathew TP, Minocha A. Effectiveness of esophageal dilation in relieving nonobstructive esophageal dysphagia and improving quality of life. South Med J 2004;97(2):137–40.

Moving?

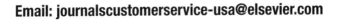

Make sure your subscription moves with you!

To notify us of your new address, find your **Clinics Account Number** (located on your mailing label above your name), and contact customer service at:

Email: journalscustomerservice-usa@elsevier.com

800-654-2452 (subscribers in the U.S. & Canada)
314-447-8871 (subscribers outside of the U.S. & Canada)

Fax number: 314-447-8029

Elsevier Health Sciences Division
Subscription Customer Service
3251 Riverport Lane
Maryland Heights, MO 63043

*To ensure uninterrupted delivery of your subscription, please notify us at least 4 weeks in advance of move.

Printed and bound by CPI Group (UK) Ltd, Croydon, CR0 4YY

03/10/2024

01040483-0017